MW00425791

CHEMOTHERAPY AND BIOTHERAPY CASE STUDIES

Edited by
Martha Polovich, PhD, RN, AOCN®
Marlon Garzo Saria, MSN, RN, AOCNS®, FAAN

Oncology Nursing Society
Pittsburgh, Pennsylvania

ONS Publications Department
Publisher and Director of Publications: William A. Tony, BA, CQIA
Managing Editor: Lisa M. George, BA
Assistant Managing Editor: Amy Nicoletti, BA, JD
Acquisitions Editor: John Zaphyr, BA, MEd
Copy Editors: Vanessa Kattouf, BA, Andrew Petyak, BA
Graphic Designer: Dany Sjoen
Editorial Assistant: Judy Holmes

Library of Congress Cataloging-in-Publication Data
Chemotherapy and biotherapy case studies / edited by Martha Polovich, Marlon Garzo Saria.
    p. ; cm.
Includes bibliographical references.
ISBN 978-1-935864-61-5
I. Polovich, Martha, editor. II. Saria, Marlon Garzo, editor. III. Oncology Nursing Society, issuing body.
    [DNLM: 1. Oncology Nursing–methods–Case Reports. 2. Antineoplastic Agents–therapeutic use–Case Reports. 3. Biological Therapy–nursing–Case Reports. 4. Drug-Related Side Effects and Adverse Reactions–nursing–Case Reports. 5. Neoplasms–drug therapy–Case Reports. 6. Neoplasms--nursing–Case Reports. WY 156]
    RM263
    615.5'8–dc23

                                                                        2015019344

Publisher's Note
This book is published by the Oncology Nursing Society (ONS). ONS neither represents nor guarantees that the practices described herein will, if followed, ensure safe and effective patient care. The recommendations contained in this book reflect ONS's judgment regarding the state of general knowledge and practice in the field as of the date of publication. The recommendations may not be appropriate for use in all circumstances. Those who use this book should make their own determinations regarding specific safe and appropriate patient care practices, taking into account the personnel, equipment, and practices available at the hospital or other facility at which they are located. The editors and publisher cannot be held responsible for any liability incurred as a consequence from the use or application of any of the contents of this book. Figures and tables are used as examples only. They are not meant to be all-inclusive, nor do they represent endorsement of any particular institution by ONS. Mention of specific products and opinions related to those products do not indicate or imply endorsement by ONS. Websites mentioned are provided for information only; the hosts are responsible for their own content and availability. Unless otherwise indicated, dollar amounts reflect U.S. dollars.
    ONS publications are originally published in English. Publishers wishing to translate ONS publications must contact ONS about licensing arrangements. ONS publications cannot be translated without obtaining written permission from ONS. (Individual tables and figures that are reprinted or adapted require additional permission from the original source.) Because translations from English may not always be accurate or precise, ONS disclaims any responsibility for inaccuracies in words or meaning that may occur as a result of the translation. Readers relying on precise information should check the original English version.

Printed in the United States of America

Integrity • Innovation • Stewardship • Advocacy • Excellence • Inclusiveness

Contributors

Editors

Martha Polovich, PhD, RN, AOCN®
Assistant Professor
Byrdine F. Lewis School of Nursing
Georgia State University
Atlanta, Georgia

Marlon Garzo Saria, MSN, RN, AOCNS®, FAAN
Neuro-Oncology Program Nurse Specialist
University of California, San Diego Medical Center – Moores Cancer Center
La Jolla, California
Case 13. Desensitization

Authors

Kristine Deano Abueg, RN, MSN, OCN®, CBCN®
Clinical Research Nurse in Oncology
Kaiser Permanente
Roseville, California
Case 4. Side Effects of Biotherapy—Oral Therapy

Amy S. Boswell, MSN, RN, OCN®
Director, Clinical Affiliations
Duke Cancer Network
Durham, North Carolina
Case 6. Cellular Therapy

Joshua Carter, BSN, RN
RN Case Manager
University of California, San Diego Medical Center – Moores Cancer Center
La Jolla, California
Case 13. Desensitization

Seth Eisenberg, RN, ASN, OCN®, BMTCN™
Professional Practice Coordinator, Infusion Services
Seattle, Washington
Case 12. Infusion Reaction

Nakia Gilliam, RN, BSN, OCN®
Clinical Nurse III
University of California, San Diego Medical Center – Moores Cancer Center
La Jolla, California
Case 2. Drug Development and Clinical Trials

Patricia Jakel, RN, MN, AOCN®
Clinical Nurse Specialist – Solid Tumor Program
UCLA Medical Center, Santa Monica
Santa Monica, California
Case 9. Oral Chemotherapy

iii

Carol S. Leija, MSN, RN, OCN®
Nursing Department Manager/Leader
  Oncology/Medical-Surgical
Kaiser Permanente
Roseville, California
Case 5. Side Effects of Biotherapy—
  Cytokine Release Syndrome

Daniel A. MacManus, RN, MSN, MBA,
  OCN®, CCRC
Clinical Nurse III
University of California, San Diego Medical
  Center – Moores Cancer Center
La Jolla, California
Case 14. Extravasation

Kathy Mooney, MSN, APRN-CNS, OCN®,
  BMTCN™
Clinical Nurse Specialist
Sidney Kimmel Comprehensive Cancer
  Center at Johns Hopkins
Baltimore, Maryland
Case 1. Bone Marrow Transplant; Case 16.
  Nausea and Vomiting

Lisa S. Moss, ANP-C, MSN, AOCNP®
Adult Nurse Practitioner
Virginia Commonwealth University
VCU Community Memorial Hospital
South Hill, Virginia
Case 3. Combination Therapy; Case 18.
  Cardiotoxicity

Paula M. Muehlbauer, RN, MSN, AOCNS®
Clinical Nurse Specialist/Academic Educa-
  tor
VA San Diego Healthcare System
San Diego, California
Case 7. Ethical Issues; Case 21. Care of
  Patient Receiving a Complicated Regi-
  men

MiKaela Olsen, MS, APRN-CNS, AOCNS®
Oncology Clinical Nurse Specialist
Sidney Kimmel Comprehensive Cancer
  Center at Johns Hopkins
Baltimore, Maryland
Case 10. Vascular Access

Syndal Ortman, APRN, DNP, FNP-BC
Nurse Practitioner; Director of Survivorship
  and Cancer Rehabilitation Programs
Hennepin County Medical Center
Minneapolis, Minnesota
Case 20. Survivorship Care Planning

Patrice E. Roberts, RN, BSN, OCN®
Oncology Staff Nurse
Sidney Kimmel Comprehensive Cancer
  Center at Johns Hopkins
Baltimore, Maryland
Case 10. Vascular Access

Madhusree Singh, MD
Associate Clinical Professor of Medicine
University of California at San Diego
  School of Medicine
VA San Diego Healthcare System
San Diego, California
Case 7. Ethical Issues

Michael Smart, RN, BSN, OCN®
Nurse Educator
Huntsville Hospital
Huntsville, Alabama
Case 8. Chemotherapy Safety; Case 11.
  Patient Assessment and Dose Calcula-
  tion

Marjorie Weiman, RN, MSN, CPHON®
Clinical Nurse Specialist, Pediatric Bone
  and Soft Tissue Sarcoma Program
UCLA Mattel Children's Hospital
Los Angeles, California
Case 19. Reproductive Toxicity

Barbara J. Wilson, MS, RN, AOCN®,
  ACNS-BC
Director, Oncology Professional Practice
WellStar Kennestone Regional Medical
  Center
Marietta, Georgia
Case 15. Myelosuppression; Case 17.
  Renal Toxicity

Disclosure

Editors and authors of books and guidelines provided by the Oncology Nursing Society are expected to disclose to the readers any significant financial interest or other relationships with the manufacturer(s) of any commercial products.

A vested interest may be considered to exist if a contributor is affiliated with or has a financial interest in commercial organizations that may have a direct or indirect interest in the subject matter. A "financial interest" may include, but is not limited to, being a shareholder in the organization; being an employee of the commercial organization; serving on an organization's speakers bureau; or receiving research funding from the organization. An "affiliation" may be holding a position on an advisory board or some other role of benefit to the commercial organization. Vested interest statements appear in the front matter for each publication.

Contributors are expected to disclose any unlabeled or investigational use of products discussed in their content. This information is acknowledged solely for the information of the readers.

The contributors provided the following disclosure and vested interest information:

Martha Polovich, PhD, RN, AOCN®: BD Medical, honoraria and other remuneration

Marlon Garzo Saria, MSN, RN, AOCNS®, FAAN: San Diego Brain Tumor Foundation, leadership position; ICU Medical, honoraria; Daisy Foundation, research funding

Seth Eisenberg, RN, ASN, OCN®, BMTCN™: Equashield Medical, CareFusion, Covidien, Corvida, consultant or advisory role; CareFusion, Takeda, Salveo Health Communications, honoraria

Patricia Jakel, RN, MN, AOCN®: Merck, Genentech, honoraria and consultant or advisory role

MiKaela Olsen, MS, APRN-CNS, AOCNS®: Equashield Medical, consultant or advisory role

Michael Smart, RN, BSN, OCN®: Equashield Medical, consultant or advisory role

Barbara J. Wilson, MS, RN, AOCN®, ACNS-BC: Amgen, honoraria

Table of Contents

Bone Marrow Transplant

Kathy Mooney, MSN, APRN-CNS, OCN®, BMTCN™

A 46-year-old man with chronic lymphocytic leukemia

R.H. is a 46-year-old man who was diagnosed with chronic lymphocytic leukemia in April 2009 and was initially treated with rituximab, cyclophosphamide, vincristine, and prednisone. A year later, his disease progressed, and he was treated with six cycles of pentostatin, cyclophosphamide, and rituximab. He presented in January 2014 with back pain, and a magnetic resonance imaging scan showed a bulky 10 cm periaortic mass with extensive disease in the abdomen. A biopsy of this mass confirmed transformation to large cell lymphoma. R.H. is now in complete remission after three cycles of bendamustine and rituximab. He is admitted to the blood and marrow transplant (BMT) unit in July for a myeloablative bone marrow transplant with a matched unrelated donor. The preparative or conditioning regimen is

- Busulfan 1 mg/kg PO on days –6 through –3
- Cyclophosphamide 50 mg/kg IV on days –2 and –1
- Cyclophosphamide 50 mg/kg IV on days +3 and +4 for graft-versus-host disease (GVHD) prophylaxis post-transplant.

On admission, R.H.'s laboratory values are all within normal limits. He has no other significant past medical history. He denies smoking and alcohol or illicit substance use. His pretransplant workup is unremarkable.

What early complication of transplant should the nurse be aware of when admitting R.H., based on his past history and transplant plan?

Veno-occlusive disease (VOD), also called sinusoidal obstruction syndrome, is the most common hepatic complication in the immediate post-transplant period and one of the most common causes of death after transplant (Sosa, 2012). The incidence of VOD is approximately 30%, with mortality as high as 70% (Anderson-Reitz & Clancy, 2013). GVHD prophylaxis using methotrexate can increase the risk. Other risk factors for VOD include (Anderson-Reitz & Clancy, 2013; Sosa, 2012)

- Prior liver impairment
- Older age
- Pretransplant chemotherapy
- Abdominal radiation
- Elevated transaminases prior to conditioning
- Allogeneic transplant
- Mismatched or unrelated donors
- Myeloablative conditioning regimens using busulfan, total body irradiation, and cyclophosphamide.

What are the signs and symptoms of veno-occlusive disease?

Two sets of diagnostic criteria are widely used for VOD: the Baltimore criteria and the Seattle criteria. The Baltimore criteria include serum bilirubin equal to or greater than 2 mg/dl within 21 days of transplantation and two of the following: enlarged liver, ascites, or weight gain of at least a 5% increase from baseline. The Seattle criteria include at least two of the following within 20 days of transplant: serum bilirubin greater than 2 mg/dl, enlarged liver or right upper quadrant pain, or sudden weight gain greater than 2% from baseline due to fluid retention (Sosa, 2012).

During R.H.'s preparative regimen, the busulfan dose is increased once based on the kinetics that were drawn with the first dose. He has no other complications during the preparative regimen. In the first week following the transplant, R.H.'s alanine transaminase and aspartate transaminase become elevated, and he complains of nausea, diarrhea, and diffuse abdominal pain. Between days 11 and 14 after his transplant, R.H.'s total bilirubin is elevated at 2.8 mg/dl, his abdomen is distended, he complains of bloating and cramping, and his weight has increased 4 kg (8.8 lbs) since admission.

How is veno-occlusive disease diagnosed?

The diagnosis of VOD is based on clinical symptoms that follow the Baltimore criteria or the Seattle criteria, as well as Doppler ultrasound of the liver that indicates reversed portal flow (Anderson-

Reitz & Clancy, 2013; Sosa, 2012). The BMT nurse should be aware of these signs and symptoms to aid in the early detection of VOD.

On day 15, R.H. is diagnosed with VOD after an ultrasound shows reversal of flow in the portal vein. On this day, his weight is up 6 kg since admission. In the following weeks, R.H.'s total serum bilirubin peaks at 41.5 mg/dl, and his creatinine peaks at 7.2 mg/dl, requiring continuous venovenous hemodialysis. He has mental status changes and respiratory failure requiring ventilator support.

What are the nursing interventions when caring for someone with suspected or confirmed veno-occlusive disease?

It is extremely important for the BMT nurse to understand the risk factors as well as the signs and symptoms of VOD to aid in early identification of patients with VOD. The RN should monitor liver function tests and coagulation studies, monitor the patient's weight for sudden increases, and accurately record intake and output. The RN should also assess for abdominal pain and edema (Sosa, 2012). After a patient has a suspected or confirmed diagnosis of VOD, it is imperative that the RN continues to monitor the patient's weight twice daily, monitor the abdominal girth, evaluate and treat pain and nausea, and monitor the patient's mental status and reorient as needed. The patient's safety should be assessed frequently because of the potential for changes in mental status. The RN should also survey the patient's environment to ensure safety (Anderson-Reitz & Clancy, 2013). Patients should be on bleeding precautions, as coagulopathy often occurs with VOD. The RN should also be aware of medications that could be potentially harmful to patients when liver enzymes or bilirubin are elevated and communicate these findings to the team (Sosa, 2012).

What is the treatment for veno-occlusive disease?

At this time, no U.S. Food and Drug Administration–approved treatments exist for VOD. Supportive measures are extremely important in the care of these patients. Mild VOD can resolve on its own, but moderate to severe VOD will require supportive interventions, such as diuretics, fluid restrictions, blood transfusion, paracentesis, and potential treatment of multi-organ failure (Sosa, 2012). Treatment should focus on managing the symptoms of VOD. Patients should be on strict fluid management to minimize intravascular and extravascular fluid overload (Anderson-Reitz & Clancy,

2013). Patients' renal function should be assessed frequently, and providers should look for ways to reduce renal injury, such as renal dosing medications and avoiding nephrotoxic agents. Acute renal failure can occur and may require hemodialysis or continuous venovenous hemodialysis (Anderson-Reitz & Clancy, 2013). Patients may require opioids for pain management, with fentanyl being the drug of choice because of its limited hepatic metabolism. Ascites and pleural effusions can be managed with paracentesis or thoracentesis; however, these procedures have their own risks, including bleeding and post-procedure hypotension due to fluid shifts. Patients have the potential for bleeding and may require frequent platelet and factor transfusions (Anderson-Reitz & Clancy, 2013).

What teaching related to veno-occlusive disease should the RN provide to patients and family members?

Prior to transplant, the RN should include education about VOD when discussing the transplant course and potential side effects of the preparative regimen. The patient should be aware of the risk of developing VOD and be willing to proceed with the transplant course (Anderson-Reitz & Clancy, 2013). Patients who exhibit signs and symptoms of VOD or who have been diagnosed with VOD should be educated about how VOD is diagnosed and treated and the importance of reporting signs and symptoms to the nurse and providers. Patients and families should be taught about bleeding precautions, including signs and symptoms of bleeding to report. Families should be informed about the signs and symptoms of mental status changes so they can report findings to the nurse. The family should be given information about support available to them, such as social workers and chaplains, as they navigate this potentially difficult time (Sosa, 2012).

Key Points

- VOD is the most common hepatic complication in the immediate post-transplant period and one of the most common causes of death after transplant.
- Two widely accepted criteria are used to diagnose VOD: the Baltimore criteria and the Seattle criteria.
- The BMT RN has an extremely important role in identifying and monitoring symptoms of VOD and needs to be skilled in symptom management.

- Patient and family education related to VOD should begin prior to the transplant and continue throughout the transplant process.

Conclusion

BMT nurses have a very important role in identifying and treating VOD. Nurses are often the first to be aware of the subtle changes that can occur in patients that lead to a diagnosis of VOD. It is imperative that all BMT nurses are aware of the signs and symptoms of VOD so that they can report these to the providers if they occur. BMT nurses also need to be aware of how important symptom management is in the treatment of VOD so that patients remain safe and comfortable during this time. Finally, BMT nurses should ensure that patients and families receive education about the risk of VOD, as well as the signs and symptoms of VOD and treatment options.

References

Anderson-Reitz, L., & Clancy, C. (2013). Hepatorenal complications. In S. Ezzone (Ed.), *Hematopoietic stem cell transplantation: A manual for nursing practice* (2nd ed., pp. 191–199). Pittsburgh, PA: Oncology Nursing Society.

Sosa, E.C. (2012). Veno-occlusive disease in hematopoietic stem cell transplantation recipients. *Clinical Journal of Oncology Nursing, 16*, 507–513. doi:10.1188/12.CJON.507-513

Oncology nurses evaluate patient outcomes and conduct research, use evidence-based practice, and/or perform continuous quality improvement studies to enhance patient care. Just as it is important for physicians to use evidence-based guidelines in managing the care of their patients, oncology nurses are equally accountable in using data-informed interventions in caring for their patients. A recent qualitative study found that the use of evidence-based practice can potentially have positive effects, including higher nurse satisfaction and retention, which could lead to cost savings for the healthcare system and improved patient care (Fridman & Frederickson, 2014).

The Oncology Nursing Society (ONS) Putting Evidence Into Practice (PEP) initiative has developed guidelines to address issues such as anxiety, pain, fatigue, nausea, and vomiting. The interventions have been rated based on likeliness to be effective and color-coded. For example, interventions with evidence to support the intervention are coded green for "go"; interventions with insufficient supporting evidence are coded yellow for "caution"; and interventions with evidence to support that they are either ineffective or may cause harm are coded red for "stop." (ONS, n.d.). Oncology nurses should refer to these guidelines when making symptom management recommendations to patients and families (ONS, n.d.).

Key Points

Evidence-based practice can have positive effects such as
- Improved patient outcomes
- Increased nurse satisfaction and retention
- Potential cost savings.

B.T. is scheduled to receive cycle 3 of six planned cycles of therapy on Tuesday and calls the clinic on Monday to "reschedule" her treatment. She leaves a message stating she has a family reunion to attend over the weekend and would prefer to reschedule her infusion for the following week.

Based on current evidence, how should the nurse respond to B.T.'s request?

Given the fact that B.T. is being treated with curative intent, it is essential to discuss the importance of relative dose intensity (RDI).

RDI refers to the ratio of delivered dose intensity (total dose delivered/total time to complete therapy) to standard dose intensity. Three separate clinical trials evaluating outcomes in patients with breast cancer related to RDI have demonstrated improved overall survival and 10-year disease-free survival in patients who received an RDI greater than or equal to 85%. Because B.T. is scheduled for cycle 3, it is not possible to accurately predict potential dose-limiting toxicities that may lead to treatment delays or dose reductions for subsequent infusions. By delaying treatment for one week due to a social event, she will decrease her RDI, potentially compromising the overall benefit of treatment (Amgen, 2008).

Key Points

- It is important for oncology nurses to educate patients and clinic staff about the importance of RDI, particularly in the curative setting.
- Oncology clinics often have nonlicensed nursing staff answering phone calls and rescheduling appointments.
- Institutions should have policies in place to ensure that patients wanting to cancel or reschedule chemotherapy visits are connected with oncology nurses— preferably oncology certified nurses—who can assess their particular situations (palliative versus curative) and reason for the delay and collaborate with patients to make the best decision for their situation.

Conclusion

Patients with cancer often have limited understanding of their treatment plans and the rationale for certain actions. While oncology nurses are accustomed to educating patients and families regarding side effects and reportable symptoms, they must also be able to reinforce the rationale for the prescribed treatment plan and ongoing monitoring. Patients present with varied levels of understanding, from having researched their treatment plan extensively online to having no understanding of their treatment plan at all. Healthcare providers must assess each patient and ensure information is provided based on the patient's education level and needs.

In addition, the field of oncology changes rapidly based on the exponential growth in data generated by research. Current treatment regimens often include multiple chemotherapy and/or biotherapy drugs. It is important for oncology nurses to remain current with new agents or new indications for already approved agents, including monitoring parameters and side effect management. Oncology nurses must understand clinical practice guidelines or consensus reports, such as those developed by the American Society of Clinical Oncology, NCCN, and ONS, and to collaborate with physicians and other allied health professionals in delivering evidence-based nursing care with the goal of improving patient outcomes.

References

Amgen. (2008). Increasing awareness of relative dose intensity in an evidence-based practice. Retrieved from http://www.onsedge.com/pdf/amgenEBP.pdf

Chu, E., & DeVita, V.T., Jr. (2014). *Physicians' cancer chemotherapy drug manual.* Burlington, MA: Jones & Bartlett Learning.

Fridman, M., & Frederickson, K. (2014). Oncology nurses and the experience of participation in an evidence-based practice project. *Oncology Nursing Forum, 41,* 382–388. doi:10.1188/14.ONF.382-388

Genentech, Inc. (2013). *Perjeta® (pertuzumab)* [Package insert]. Retrieved from http://www.gene.com/gene/products/information/perjeta/pdf/perjeta_prescribing.pdf

National Comprehensive Cancer Network. (2015). *NCCN Clinical Practice Guidelines in Oncology (NCCN Guidelines®): Breast cancer* [v. 1.2015]. Retrieved from http://www.nccn.org/professionals/physician_gls/pdf/breast.pdf

Oncology Nursing Society. (n.d.). Putting evidence into practice. Retrieved from https://www.ons.org/practice-resources/pep

Polovich, M., Olsen, M., & LeFebvre, K.B. (Eds.). (2014). *Chemotherapy and biotherapy guidelines and recommendations for practice* (4th ed.). Pittsburgh, PA: Oncology Nursing Society.

CASE 4
Side Effects of Biotherapy— Oral Therapy

Kristine Deano Abueg, RN, MSN, OCN®, CBCN®

A 62-year-old woman with bilateral non-small cell lung cancer

K.J. is a 62-year-old female nonsmoker recently diagnosed with bilateral non-small cell lung cancer (NSCLC). Genomic testing reveals that her tumor harbors a mutation in the epidermal growth factor receptor (EGFR) gene. Her physician prescribes the oral tyrosine kinase inhibitor erlotinib and explains that this daily pill, taken on an empty stomach, will be the primary treatment for her lung cancer. While ordering the prescription, K.J.'s physician schedules an education session at the oral therapies clinic. K.J. is advised to fill the prescription at her local pharmacy and bring the medication to her education session.

K.J. replies that she likes the option of the oral therapy because it fits into her busy lifestyle. She also states that she is already on several oral medications and is confident that she can take the erlotinib without the need for one-on-one education.

How will one-on-one personalized education benefit this patient prior to the start of erlotinib?

Adherence, drug interactions, food interactions, and schedule complexity greatly affect the effectiveness and side effects of oral anticancer agents. Normally, patients with cancer who receive IV therapy will frequently receive in-depth oncology education while receiving their infusion. Although oral therapy may provide more treatment independence and flexibility, it reduces the opportunity for clinicians to assess and educate patients. One-on-one in-depth education provided by the nurse and consultation with the pharmacist will give K.J.'s medical team an opportunity to establish a rapport with K.J., which promotes communication, adherence, and safety (Esper, 2013; Lester, 2012; Moody & Jackowski, 2010; Neuss et al., 2013; Schneider, Hess, & Gosselin, 2011; Winkeljohn, 2010). Specific items to discuss at this initial meeting include the following: (1) importance of treatment adherence, (2) safe handling, (3) detailed instruction on dosing schedule, (4) symptom management of key side effects, (5) current medication reconciliation and drug and food interactions, (6) plan for missed doses, and (7) healthcare provider contact information (Esper, 2013; Lester, 2012; Neuss et al., 2013; Winkeljohn, 2010). The nurse plans to access the Oncology Nursing Society's *Tools for Oral Adherence Toolkit* for useful resources (www.ons.org/sites/default/files/oral%20adherence%20toolkit.pdf).

Key Points

- A shift to oral therapies requires that the healthcare team develop alternative methods for patient monitoring and education other than those traditionally offered during parenteral therapy visits.
- Key elements of oral medication education should include written and verbal instructions on
  - Intent of the therapy, including a discussion on diagnosis, therapy goals, and planned duration of treatment
  - Discussion on the importance of treatment adherence to side effect management and efficacy
  - Safe handling education
  - Detailed instructions on dosing schedule
  - Symptom management of key side effects
  - Current medication reconciliation and drug and food interactions
  - Plan for missed doses
  - Healthcare provider contact information.

What assessments by the nurse will promote adherence?

An assessment of the patient's coping abilities and identification of any barriers to adherence are important first steps (Schneider et al., 2011). Barriers to adherence include psychosocial coping issues, financial barriers, regimen complexity, availability of patient resources, and side effect management. Patients who are anxious or frightened or who have negative beliefs about the value of therapy are unlikely to absorb information adequately and may be less willing to adhere to an effective dosing schedule (Moore, 2007). Healthcare providers should explore financial constraints, as insurance coverage limitations can vary greatly and affect patients' ability to fill prescriptions (Esper, 2013). Once barriers are identified, the nurse should tailor the patient education using appropriate written and verbal communication, rather than scripted dialogue, with sufficient opportunity for the patient to ask questions and reflect understanding and engagement (Neuss et al., 2013). Patient-tailored techniques help ensure the doses are taken at the appropriate time (Esper, 2013; Moore, 2007; Schneider et al., 2011). The patient's family members and/or caregivers should also be invited to attend. These steps will help to develop a rapport and trust between K.J. and her providers, which will in turn facilitate communication and willingness to learn (Winkeljohn, 2010).

K.J. attends the oral chemotherapy initiation teaching. At the appointment, the nurse provides a pill calendar so K.J. can document the time of each dose. Written instructions are printed prominently at the top of each page of the calendar. Written and verbal instructions include the name (both generic and brand name) of the drug, how many pills per dose, how many doses per day, and what times to take each dose (Winkeljohn, 2010). Additionally, the nurse instructs K.J. to avoid drug-drug and drug-food reactions.

The nurse reviews the medication instructions:
- Take erlotinib (150 mg) once a day on an empty stomach. An empty stomach means at least one hour before and/or two hours after food or drink (other than water). See Figure 4-1 for examples of dosing schedules with respect to meals/snacks.
- Do not start any new medications until it has been reviewed by your healthcare team. Oral anticancer drugs may cause negative reactions when mixed with other medications.
- Side effects of erlotinib can include skin changes. Consult immediately with your healthcare team if you start to experience any skin or nail changes.
- On each calendar day, indicate when the dose was taken and the time of last food prior to dose.

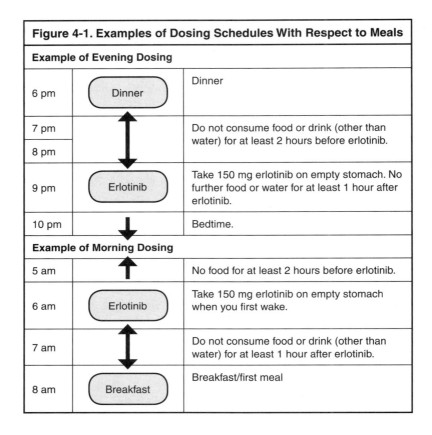

Figure 4-1. Examples of Dosing Schedules With Respect to Meals

Example of Evening Dosing

6 pm	Dinner	Dinner
7 pm		Do not consume food or drink (other than water) for at least 2 hours before erlotinib.
8 pm		
9 pm	Erlotinib	Take 150 mg erlotinib on empty stomach. No further food or water for at least 1 hour after erlotinib.
10 pm		Bedtime.

Example of Morning Dosing

5 am		No food for at least 2 hours before erlotinib.
6 am	Erlotinib	Take 150 mg erlotinib on empty stomach when you first wake.
7 am		Do not consume food or drink (other than water) for at least 1 hour after erlotinib.
8 am	Breakfast	Breakfast/first meal

What teaching about safe handling should the nurse provide to K.J. at this time?

Oral anticancer agents require special handling and disposal to minimize exposure of caregivers and the environment. Oral anticancer agents should not be disposed of in the regular trash, nor should they be flushed down the drain or toilet. According to the National Institute for Occupational Safety and Health, American Society of Clinical Oncology, and Oncology Nursing Society, oral anticancer agents should be handled with the same caution as parenteral agents (Neuss et al., 2013). The nurse tells K.J. that body fluids, such as urine, fecal matter, blood, or vomit, can be contaminated with chemotherapy. She should wash any body fluid–soiled linen separately from other laundry. Figure 4-2 lists key recommendations about safe handling.

After two weeks of therapy, the nurse initiates a follow-up call to K.J. The patient reports she is tolerating treatment generally well, but that she has noticed she tends to get an upset stomach. In the past, she has taken an over-the-counter antacid, and she wants to start taking one to combat stomach discomfort.

What instruction should the nurse provide regarding concomitant medication and food?

Because adverse events can contribute to decreased adherence, the nurse assesses the character, timing, and impact on quality of life. The nurse asks when the discomfort begins in relationship to

---

Figure 4-2. Safe Handling of Oral Chemotherapy

Storage
- Do not store medications in areas where food or drinks are stored or consumed.
- Do not leave medication in open areas, near sources of water, in direct sunlight, or where they can be accessed by children or pets.

Disposal
- Do not discard medication down the drain or toilet or in the garbage.
- Retain all wet, damaged, unused, discontinued, or expired medications in a tightly sealed plastic bag. Store this bag securely away from other trash, food, and medication. Contact your pharmacist or clinic for disposal instructions.

Body Fluids
- Body fluids include sweat, vomit, urine, fecal matter, and blood.
- Linen that has been in contact with any body fluids should be considered contaminated.
- Wash any soiled linen separately from other laundry items.

Handling
- Limit the number of individuals who come in contact with the medication.
- Transport and store medicine as instructed and as outlined in the packaging label. On receiving your prescription, review the package label, specifically checking medication name and dosage.
- Do not break, crush, open, or manipulate the pill in any way, as this may result in unintended exposure.
- Use gloves, if possible, and wash hands thoroughly before and after glove application. If gloves are not worn, tip tablets and capsules from their container/blister pack directly into a disposable medicine cup. Contact your pharmacist or clinic for disposal instructions.

Note. Based on information from Goodin et al., 2011; Lester, 2012; Neuss et al., 2013; Polovich, 2011.

food or pill intake; if the discomfort is associated with any other symptoms such as vomiting, diarrhea, constipation, or pain; and if these symptoms affect her sleep or daily activities. Drug-drug interactions are more common with oral agents than parenteral medications, so limiting adverse interactions is an important aspect of managing oral therapies. The nurse reinforces that K.J. should not start any medication (over-the-counter, herbal, or prescription) without consulting her physician. Erlotinib is affected by changes in gastric pH, so acid-reducing agents can adversely affect the target dosing. Proton pump inhibitors are contraindicated. K.J. can take an antacid as long as it and the erlotinib are separated by several hours. If an antacid alone is ineffective, the physician may consider an H_2 receptor antagonist such as ranitidine. Erlotinib should be taken no less than 10 hours after the H_2 receptor antagonist or two hours before the next dose of the H_2 receptor antagonist (see Table 4-1).

Five weeks after the beginning of therapy, K.J. returns to the clinic for a follow-up assessment. She is tolerating the treatment well overall, but she has a rash.

What should the nurse assess regarding the rash?

To thoroughly assess the rash, the nurse asks when it first occurred, which body areas are involved, and whether it is itchy. K.J. reports that

Table 4-1. Interactions Between Gastric Acid–Reducing Agents and Erlotinib

Acid Suppressive Compound	Effective Action on Concentration of Erlotinib	Dosing Recommendation
Proton pump inhibitors: Omeprazole 40 mg daily	Decrease by 46%	Do not use.
H_2 receptor antagonist: Ranitidine 150 mg twice daily	Decrease by 15%	Take erlotinib 10 hours after H_2 receptor antagonist and at least 2 hours before.
Antacids	Not yet evaluated	Separate dose from erlotinib by several hours.

Note. Based on information from OSI Pharmaceuticals, 2014; van Leeuwen et al., 2014.

the rash began about two weeks ago on her chest and face. It started as dry skin, then it began to look like acne. She has not had a fever or drainage, but K.J. reports itching and admits to scratching. If the rash had had drainage, the nurse would obtain cultures to rule out secondary bacterial infection and identify appropriate antibiotic therapy.

Because EGFR rash is frequently associated with other dermatologic changes, the nurse also assesses for hair and nail changes. Rashes can negatively affect quality of life, so patients may be prone to discontinue or reduce doses prematurely. Thus, the nurse explores the impact on K.J.'s emotional well-being and coping ability. Treatment of EGFR rash is based on associated symptoms and grading of severity (see Table 4-2). After assessing the severity, the nurse consults with the multidisciplinary team to formulate an appropriate action plan.

What education about EGFR rash is especially important?

EGFR rash is a significant cause of morbidity, leading to interruption of drug therapy (Lacouture et al., 2011). The nurse advises K.J. that the development and severity of the rash have been associated with better clinical outcomes and longer survival (Liu et al., 2013; Wacker et al., 2007). K.J. is counseled on the usual cyclic pattern of EGFR rash. The rash cycle typically appears within the first two weeks of therapy, peaks at weeks four through six, and decreases in severity after weeks six through eight. After week eight, the rash often recurs with the same pattern (Lacouture et al., 2011). The rash can look like acne, causing patients to try over-the-counter acne treatments (Lacouture, Basti, Patel, & Benson, 2006; Lacouture et al., 2011). The nurse advises K.J. to avoid these acne-directed preparations, as they may exacerbate skin sensitivity. The nurse also encourages K.J. to use sun protection, avoid trauma, and apply alcohol-free moisturizers twice daily to the entire body (Lacouture et al., 2006, 2011; Melosky, 2012; Wacker et al., 2007). Additionally, the nurse advises K.J. that skin changes, including erythema and hyperpigmentation, can persist after resolution of pustules. Early interventions, including patient education, self-care techniques, and prompt reporting of symptoms, are important steps to minimize late effects and promote treatment continuation (Lacouture et al., 2011).

Table 4-2. Epidermal Growth Factor Receptor Inhibitor–Induced Rash Assessment and Treatment Recommendations

Severity	Presentation	Treatment Options
None (prevention)	No rash or skin changes	Avoid sun and use sunscreen (SPF 15 or higher), preferably containing zinc oxide or titanium oxide. Apply alcohol-free emollients to entire body twice daily. Avoid drying agents. Take medication on empty stomach with full glass of water.
Mild	Localized, minimal symptoms No drainage or fever Minimal impact on self-care or daily activities	Reinforce prevention strategies. Reinforce patient education and supportive care. Apply topical hydrocortisone (1% or 2.5% cream) or clindamycin (1% gel). Dose reduction is NOT recommended.
Moderate	Appearance of pustules with mild pruritus or tenderness No drainage or fever Minimal impact on self-care or daily activities	Reinforce prevention strategies. Reinforce patient education and supportive care. Apply hydrocortisone (2.5% cream), clindamycin (1% gel), or pimecrolimus (1% cream), with the addition of doxycycline (100 mg PO BID) or minocycline (100 mg PO BID). Dose reduction is NOT recommended.
Severe	Generalized rash accompanied by severe pruritus and tenderness Can be associated with drainage and/ or fever—evidence of superinfection Has impact on self-care and/or daily activities	Consider dose reduction or interruption. Reinforce prevention strategies. Reinforce patient education and supportive care. Consider addition of methylprednisolone dose pack. Apply hydrocortisone (2.5% cream), clindamycin (1% gel), or pimecrolimus (1% cream), with the addition of doxycycline (100 mg PO BID) or minocycline (100 mg PO BID).

Note. Based on information from Eaby et al., 2008; Lacouture et al., 2011; Melosky, 2012.

Drug-drug or drug-food interactions can also influence rash severity. The nurse asks K.J. to describe how she typically takes her doses. K.J. replies that she prefers to take her pills at 6:30 am when she wakes up, just before she leaves for work at 7:15 am. When asked about morning meals, K.J. replies that she tries to "grab a bite" before or during work. The nurse reminds K.J. that she should abstain from food or drink (other than water) for at least one hour after taking erlotinib because food increases bioavailability and can intensify side effects (Melosky, 2012).

The interdisciplinary team prescribes doxycycline (100 mg orally, twice daily) to control pustule inflammation and pruritus (Eaby, Culkin, & Lacouture, 2008; Lacouture et al., 2011; Melosky, 2012).

Key Points

- Rash is a common side effect of anti-EGFR therapy and can be associated with a significant impact on quality of life.
- Rash severity has been associated with EGFR efficacy.
- Patients should be taught self-care preventive techniques.
- Treatment is based on assessment of severity.
- Drug-drug and drug-food interactions affect drug bioavailability and can intensify side effects.

At a follow-up assessment two weeks later, K.J. reports that some scarring remains but that itching has decreased. She remains on erlotinib therapy at the full dose.

Conclusion

K.J., a 62-year-old woman diagnosed with EGFR-overexpressing, metastatic NSCLC, is prescribed the oral tyrosine kinase inhibitor erlotinib. The patient receives thorough education regarding dose schedule, safe handling, and adherence. Soon after initiating therapy, K.J. reports heartburn and is counseled on the safe management of her symptoms while avoiding adverse drug reactions. Several weeks into therapy, K.J. reports symptoms consistent with expected EGFR inhibitor–associated rash. She is counseled on rash management techniques and prescribed an oral tetracycline. She remains on the full erlotinib dose, employing preventive strategies to manage side effects.

References

Eaby, B., Culkin, A., & Lacouture, M.E. (2008). An interdisciplinary consensus on managing skin reactions associated with human epidermal growth factor inhibitors. *Clinical Journal of Oncology Nursing, 12,* 283–290. doi:10.1188/08.CJON.283-290

Esper, P. (2013). Identifying strategies to optimize care with oral cancer therapy. *Clinical Journal of Oncology Nursing, 17,* 629–636. doi:10.1188/13.CJON.629-636

Goodin, S., Griffith, N., Chen, B., Chuk, K., Daouphars, M., Doreau, C., ... Meier, K. (2011). Safe handling of oral chemotherapeutic agents in clinical practice: Recommendations from an international pharmacy panel. *Journal of Oncology Practice, 7,* 7–12. doi:10.1200/JOP.2010.000068

Lacouture, M.E., Basti, S., Patel, J., & Benson, A. (2006). The SERIES clinic: An interdisciplinary approach to the management of toxicities of EGFR inhibitors. *Journal of Supportive Oncology, 4,* 236–238.

Lacouture, M.E., Anadkat, M.J., Bedsadoun, R.-J., Bryce, J., Chan, A., Epstein, J.B., ... Murphy, B.A. (2011). Clinical practice guidelines for the prevention and treatment of EGFR inhibitor-associated dermatological toxicities. *Supportive Care in Cancer, 19,* 1079–1095. doi:10.1007/s00520-011-1197-6

Lester, J. (2012). Safe handling and administration considerations of oral anticancer agents in the clinical and home setting [Online exclusive]. *Clinical Journal of Oncology Nursing, 16,* E192–E197. doi:10.1188/12.CJON.E192-E197

Liu, H.B., Wu, Y., Lv, T.F., Yao, Y.W., Xiao, Y.Y., Yuan, D.M., & Song, Y. (2013). Skin rash could predict the response to EGFR tyrosine kinase inhibitor and the prognosis for patients with non-small cell lung cancer: A systematic review and meta-analysis. *PLOS ONE, 8,* e55128. doi:10.1371/journal.pone.0055128

Melosky, B. (2012). Supportive care treatments for toxicities of anti-EGFR and other targeted agents. *Current Oncology, 19*(Suppl. 1), S59–S63. doi:10.3747/co.19.1054

Moody, M., & Jackowski, J. (2010). Are your patients on oral chemotherapy in your practice setting safe? *Clinical Journal of Oncology Nursing, 14,* 339–346. doi:10.1188/10.CJON.339-346

Moore, S. (2007). Facilitating oral chemotherapy compliance through patient/family-focused education. *Cancer Nursing, 30,* 112–122. doi:10.1097/01.NCC.0000265009.33053.2d

Neuss, M.N., Polovich, M., McNiff, K., Esper, P., Gilmore, T.R., LeFebvre, K.B., ... Jacobson, J.O. (2013). 2013 updated American Society of Clinical Oncology/Oncology Nursing Society chemotherapy administration safety standards including standards for the safe administration and management of oral chemotherapy. *Journal of Oncology Practice, 9*(Suppl. 2), 5s–13s. doi:10.1200/JOP.2013.000874

OSI Pharmaceuticals. (2014). *Tarceva® (erlotinib)* [Package insert]. Northbrook, IL: Author.

Polovich, M. (Ed.). (2011). *Safe handling of hazardous drugs* (2nd ed.). Pittsburgh, PA: Oncology Nursing Society.

Schneider, S.M., Hess, K., & Gosselin, T. (2011). Interventions to promote adherence with oral agents. *Seminars in Oncology Nursing, 27,* 133–141. doi:10.1016/j.soncn.2011.02.005

van Leeuwen, R.W., van Gelder, T., Mathijssen, R.H., & Jansman, F.G. (2014). Drug-drug interactions with tyrosine kinase inhibitors: A clinical perspective. *Lancet Oncology, 15,* e315–e326. doi:10.1016/S1470-2045(13)70579-5

Wacker, B., Nagrani, T., Wienberg, J., Witt, K., Clark, G., & Cagnoni, P.J. (2007). Correlation between development of rash and efficacy in patients treated with the epidermal growth factor receptor tyrosine kinase inhibitor erlotinib in two large phase III studies. *Clinical Cancer Research, 13,* 3913–3921. doi:10.1158/1078-0432.CCR-06-2610

Winkeljohn, D. (2010). Adherence of oral cancer therapies. *Clinical Journal of Oncology Nursing, 14,* 461–466. doi:10.1188/10.CJON.461-466

CASE 5
Side Effects of Biotherapy— Cytokine Release Syndrome

Carol S. Leija, MSN, RN, OCN®

A 71-year-old man receiving a monoclonal antibody

R.Y. is a 71-year-old man who presents to the emergency department with abdominal pain accompanied by a poor appetite. During further nursing assessment, R.Y. reports that he has been experiencing frequent night sweats, recent weight loss, and fatigue. R.Y.'s past medical history includes ureteral stent placement and a history of coronary artery bypass graft. The physician's physical assessment notes a large abdominal mass. Further radiologic examination reveals a 12 × 13 × 18 cm irregularly shaped abdominal mass with nearby sites of hypermetabolic adenopathy in the liver and celiac axis. A retroperitoneal lymph node biopsy is obtained and reveals diffuse large B-cell lymphoma, Ann Arbor stage III.

Diffuse large B-cell lymphoma is a neoplasm that arises from mature B cells. This non-Hodgkin lymphoma is the most common lymphoid malignant disease. It will often manifest with a rapidly growing nodal or extranodal mass, with the most common sites being the bone marrow and gastrointestinal tract. Patients often report unexplained weight loss, fever, and drenching night sweats, commonly known as B symptoms (Goodrich, McNally, Ridgeway, & Zitella, 2013). Because of the aggressive nature of the disease, urgent treatment is recommended (Long, 2007).

R.Y. is now admitted to the inpatient oncology unit for induction chemotherapy and biotherapy for treatment of non-Hodgkin lymphoma. The oncologist orders the monoclonal antibody (mAb) rituximab, in combination with cyclophosphamide, doxorubicin, vincristine, and prednisone (R-CHOP), based on evidence that adding rituximab to the CHOP chemotherapy regimen increases overall response rates in non-Hodgkin lymphoma (Peranski, 2007).

Biotherapy refers to treatments derived from biologic sources that are used to modify, augment, or restore the immune system (Appel, 2007; Polovich, Olsen, & LeFebvre, 2014). Biotherapy agents used today include hematopoietic growth factors, interleukins, vaccines, interferons, and mAbs. The mAbs may be derived from human, mouse, or combination human-mouse antibodies. These agents recognize the host cell as foreign and attack through a variety of targeted approaches (Polovich et al., 2014).

Rituximab is an mAb that identifies and binds to the CD20 antigen found in B-cell lymphoma cells. This antibody-antigen binding complex results in cell toxicity or death (Polovich et al., 2014). The antibody-antigen binding complex can generate a rapid release of cytokines into the bloodstream that may cause chills, fever, nausea, hypotension, and headache. These cytokine-mediated infusion reactions are common with the administration of mAbs and most often occur during the initial infusion. The nurse must be familiar with prevention and management of infusion reactions to promote optimal patient outcomes.

The oncologist explains to R.Y. that his treatment plan will include the R-CHOP regimen every 21 days for six to eight cycles (Genentech, Inc., 2013a), frequent monitoring of his laboratory values, ongoing diagnostic imaging, and regular physical assessments (Long, 2007). Informed consent for the combination biotherapy and chemotherapy regimen is obtained by the physician and witnessed by the nurse.

The R-CHOP protocol for cycle 1 is as follows:
- Prednisone 50 mg tabs. Two tablets taken orally daily with food for five days (first dose 30 minutes prior to rituximab on day 1).
- Rituximab 375 mg/m^2 IV on day 1. Start at 50 mg/hr and increase by 50 mg/hr every 30 minutes, if no reaction occurs, to a maximum of 400 mg/hr (Vogel, 2010).
- Doxorubicin 50 mg/m^2 IV on day 2
- Vincristine 1.4 mg/m^2 IV on day 2
- Cyclophosphamide 750 mg/m^2/day IV on day 2

What education specific to monoclonal antibodies should the nurse provide?

The nurse provides R.Y. and his family with initial education regarding his disease, treatment, symptom management, and resources for

References

Appel, C.P. (2007). Biotherapy. In M.E. Langhorne, J.S. Fulton, & S.E. Otto (Eds.), *Oncology nursing* (5th ed., pp. 377–387). St. Louis, MO: Elsevier Mosby.

Genentech, Inc. (2013a). NHL dosing. Retrieved from http://www.rituxan.com/hem/hcp/dosing/nhl-dosing

Genentech, Inc. (2013b). 90-minute infusion for previously untreated DLBCL and follicular NHL patients in cycles 2–8. Retrieved from http://www.rituxan.com/hem/hcp/dosing/nhl-dosing/90-minute-infusion

Goodrich, A., McNally, G.A, Ridgeway, J., & Zitella, L.J. (2013). Mature B-cell neoplasms. In M. Olsen & L.J. Zitella (Eds.), *Hematologic malignancies in adults* (pp. 301–361). Pittsburgh, PA: Oncology Nursing Society.

Lang, D.S.P., & Fong, C.C. (2014). Prediction of adverse events in patients receiving rapid rituximab infusion: Validation of a predictive model. *Clinical Journal of Oncology Nursing, 18*, 89–92. doi:10.1188/14.CJON.89-92

Long, J. (2007). Treatment approaches and nursing applications for non-Hodgkin lymphoma. *Clinical Journal of Oncology Nursing, 11*(Suppl. 1), 13–21. doi:10.1188/07.CJON.S1.13-21

National Cancer Institute Cancer Therapy Evaluation Program. (2010). *Common terminology criteria for adverse events* [v.4.03]. Retrieved from http://evs.nci.nih.gov/ftp1/CTCAE/CTCAE_4.03_2010-06-14_QuickReference_5x7.pdf

Peranski, K. (2007). Malignant lymphoma. In M.E. Langhorne, J.S. Fulton, & S.E. Otto (Eds.), *Oncology nursing* (5th ed., pp. 275–289). St. Louis, MO: Elsevier Mosby.

Polovich, M., Olsen, M., & LeFebvre, L.B. (Eds.). (2014). *Chemotherapy and biotherapy guidelines and recommendations for practice* (4th ed.). Pittsburgh, PA: Oncology Nursing Society.

Vogel, W.H. (2010). Infusion reactions: Diagnosis, assessment, and management [Online exclusive]. *Clinical Journal of Oncology Nursing, 14*, E10–E21. doi:10.1188/10.CJON.E10-E21

CASE 6
Cellular Therapy

Amy S. Boswell, MSN, RN, OCN®

A 71-year-old man receiving sipuleucel-T

T.F. is a 71-year-old man diagnosed with minimally symptomatic metastatic castration-resistant (hormone-refractory) prostate cancer. Eight years ago, he presented with an elevated prostate-specific antigen (PSA) test result. A subsequent prostate biopsy confirmed Gleason 6 prostate cancer with bone metastases discovered upon bone scan and confirmed via magnetic resonance imaging scan. Previous treatments for his prostate cancer include leuprolide acetate for depot suspension and bicalutamide. The patient has chronic back pain that has been well controlled with medications. After evaluating T.F.'s history, his physician prescribes sipuleucel-T.

What information needs to be included in patient education prior to beginning sipuleucel-T?

Sipuleucel-T is an autologous cellular immunotherapy indicated for patients with asymptomatic or mildly symptomatic metastatic castration-resistant prostate cancer (Dendreon Corp., 2014). When this treatment was approved by the U.S. Food and Drug Administration in April 2010, it was the first antigen-specific immunotherapy approved for cancer treatment (Drake, 2010). The randomized phase III IMPACT trial showed a median overall survival improvement of 4.1 months for sipuleucel-T compared to placebo (25.8 months versus 21.7 months, respectively). However, there was no significant effect on time to disease progression or PSA levels, and

43

most men require subsequent therapy to maintain control over disease progression (Kantoff et al., 2010).

The immunotherapy is a product of leukapheresis. Depending on the quality of an individual patient's venous access, a dual-lumen apheresis catheter may be required for central venous access prior to starting therapy. Leukapheresis involves selective removal of white blood cells and is well tolerated, although catheter complications (e.g., blood clots, infection, bleeding) have been reported. The immunotherapy is manufactured using the apheresed cells and administered intravenously three days later. This process is repeated for a total of three infusions over six weeks (dosing every two weeks). Although the treatment is generally well tolerated, possible adverse effects include fatigue, nausea, headache, joint ache, back pain, chills, and fever. If, for any reason, the patient is unable to receive a scheduled infusion, the patient will need to undergo an additional leukapheresis procedure prior to continuing a course of treatment.

What is the proposed mechanism of action for sipuleucel-T?

Three days prior to the planned infusion date, autologous CD54+ mononuclear cells are collected by leukapheresis from the patient. These cells are shipped to the manufacturer and activated in culture with prostatic acid phosphatase granulocyte macrophage–colony-stimulating factor (PAP-GM-CSF) for subsequent infusion to the patient. The activated cells are designed to induce an immune response targeted against prostatic acid phosphatase antigen expressed in patients with prostate cancer (Polovich, Olsen, & LeFebvre, 2014).

What are the considerations regarding leukapheresis?

Each dose of sipuleucel-T requires a standard leukapheresis procedure approximately three days prior to the infusion. Leukapheresis takes about three to four hours to complete. Potential adverse events that could occur during or within 24 hours of a leukapheresis procedure include oral paresthesia (tingling around the mouth), paresthesia (tingling in the fingers), dizziness, fatigue, nausea, feeling cold, and fainting. Patients should be encouraged to hydrate well and plan for someone to take them home after the procedure (Dendreon Corp., 2013a). The patient's peripheral veins must be suitable for (or must be able to accommodate) insertion of two large-bore (16- or 18-gauge) needles on the day of leukapheresis. Because leukapheresis is typically a two-arm procedure, both arms should be assessed. This assessment should be completed by a healthcare provider at least one week prior to beginning leukapheresis to allow arrangements to be made for central venous access, if required. If the patient's peripheral venous access is not adequate, placement of an apheresis catheter by an interventional radiologist or surgeon is required for central venous access prior to starting this therapy. The catheter should be a large-bore, dual-lumen, dialysis-type apheresis catheter that is able to support blood flow of greater than 50 ml/min (Dendreon Corp., 2013b).

The apheresis nurse notes that T.F. is unable to have his first leukapheresis procedure because his veins are too small. What should have been done to prevent this delay, and what should be done next?

T.F.'s bilateral peripheral veins should have been assessed by a healthcare provider (e.g., infusion nurse) prior to leukapheresis. Because the apheresis nurse has determined that T.F. has inadequate peripheral venous access, his physician, physician assistant (PA), or advanced practice nurse (APN) needs to order and schedule the insertion of an apheresis catheter by an interventional radiologist or surgeon. His leukapheresis can then be rescheduled.

What are the nursing considerations during infusion of sipuleucel-T?

Sipuleucel-T is infused intravenously over 60 minutes. To minimize potential acute infusion reactions, the patient should be premedicated orally with acetaminophen and an antihistamine, such as diphenhydramine, 30 minutes prior to infusion (per provider order). Symptoms of acute infusion reactions include fever, rigor or chills, fatigue, nausea, vomiting, respiratory events (e.g., dyspnea, hypoxia, bronchospasm), and headache or joint ache. If a reaction occurs, stop the infusion and administer appropriate medical treatment as needed (per provider or standing order). In sipuleucel-T clinical trials, symptoms were treated with acetaminophen, IV H_1 and/or H_2 blockers, and low-dose IV meperidine (Dendreon Corp., 2014). Syncope, hypotension, hypertension, and tachycardia are also potential symptoms of an acute infusion reaction, so patients with cardiac or pulmonary conditions should be closely monitored (Dendreon Corp., 2014). To maintain patient safety, the patient and family must be educated to recognize early signs of an acute infusion reaction and immediately notify the nurse in order to receive prompt management. Written protocols or standing orders for management of infusion reactions are strongly recommended to support immediate action (Vogel, 2014).

Each dose of sipuleucel-T is cellularly unique and should only be used for one specific patient. Prior to infusion, confirmation of product release using patient-specific product disposition forms must be completed. The product should not be removed from the insulated container until the time of infusion. Clinicians must use universal precautions during handling because sipuleucel-T is a cellular product. A cell filter should not be used. The product should not be administered if the bag is leaking or damaged or if clumps can be seen in the bag. Once the infusion product is removed from insulated storage, it should not remain at room temperature for longer than three hours. Also, the infusion must be completed prior to the infusion product's expiration date and time (Dendreon Corp., 2014).

T.F. complains of rigors, chills, and a headache during the last 15 minutes of his first infusion. How should the nurse manage these symptoms?

Each institution's sipuleucel-T regimen should include standing orders for an infusion reaction. The nurse immediately stops the infusion and obtains a full set of vital signs. The nurse then starts a 250 ml bolus of normal saline and notifies the physician, PA, or APN. Next, the nurse administers meperidine 25 mg IV for the rigors/chills and promethazine 12.5 mg IV (an H_1 antagonist). After about 20 minutes, T.F.'s symptoms resolve and he is cleared by the PA or APN to receive the remainder of his infusion. The infusion is restarted at the same rate, and he completes the infusion with no further issues.

During the course of his sipuleucel-T treatments, T.F. has consistently experienced fatigue. How can the nurse address these symptoms?

Over the course of three treatments, T.F.'s fatigue score has ranged between 3 and 5 on a scale of 0–10, with 10 being the worst fatigue of his life. *Cancer-related fatigue* is defined as "a distressing persistent, subjective sense of physical, emotional and/or cognitive tiredness or exhaustion related to cancer or cancer treatment that is not proportional to recent activity and interferes with usual functioning" (National Comprehensive Cancer Network®, 2015, p.

FT-1). Interventions that can improve T.F.'s fatigue include exercise, cognitive behavioral intervention, energy conservation and activity management, certain types of ginseng, management of concurrent symptoms, massage therapy, mindfulness-based stress reduction, psychoeducation, and yoga (Oncology Nursing Society, 2014).

After the nurse presented options to address his fatigue, T.F. decided to try exercise and energy conservation techniques. One research study demonstrated that ongoing exercise benefits adults in treatment for first-time prostate and other cancers. Participants who engaged in more aerobic exercise reported less fatigue than those who had engaged in less aerobic exercise. T.F. was educated that incorporating a 30-minute brisk walk five days each week could help reduce fatigue associated with cancer treatments (Wenzel et al., 2013). In a meta-analysis, exercise reduced cancer-related fatigue, especially in theory-based programs involving moderate-intensity resistance exercise among older cancer survivors (Brown et al., 2011). In a randomized clinical trial, energy conservation and activity management (ECAM) demonstrated a greater decrease in fatigue over time when compared to the control group. ECAM is used "to balance rest and activity during time of high fatigue so that valued activities and goals can be maintained" (Barsevick et al., 2004, p. 1303). Examples include delegation, priority setting, and increased time for rest.

T.F. has now successfully completed all three sipuleucel-T infusions. What further action should be taken?

The nurse should ensure that T.F. has been scheduled for the removal of his apheresis catheter as soon as possible to avoid further risk of infection or other catheter-related complications.

Conclusion

T.F. is a 71-year-old man diagnosed with metastatic hormone-refractory prostate cancer who successfully completed his sipuleucel-T treatment. As recommended, he has continued to receive leuprolide acetate 30 mg intramuscular injections every four months for medical castration (Kantoff et al., 2010). He will return to see his provider for restaging scans and treatment planning in six weeks.

Key Points

- Sipuleucel-T is an autologous cellular immunotherapy indicated for patients with asymptomatic or mildly symptomatic metastatic castration-resistant (hormone-refractory) prostate cancer prior to chemotherapy (Dendreon Corp., 2014).
- Leukapheresis is required three days prior to each treatment to obtain autologous CD54+ mononuclear cells from the patient. These cells are shipped to the manufacturer and activated in culture with PAP-GM-CSF for subsequent infusion to the patient (Polovich et al., 2014).
- Important nursing considerations include the following.
  - Peripheral venous access must be assessed at least one week prior to initial leukapheresis procedure.
  - Confirmation of product release using patient-specific product disposition forms must be completed prior to infusion.
  - Completion of infusion must occur prior to the infusion product's expiration date and time.
  - Acute infusion reaction may occur and requires prompt management.

References

Barsevick, A.M., Dudley, W., Beck, S., Sweeney, C., Whitmer, K., & Nail, L. (2004). A randomized clinical trial of energy conservation for patients with cancer-related fatigue. *Cancer, 100,* 1302–1310. doi:10.1002/cncr.20111

Brown, J.C., Huedo-Medina, T.B., Pescatello, L.S., Pescatello, S.M., Ferrer, R.A., & Johnson, B.T. (2011). Efficacy of exercise interventions in modulating cancer-related fatigue among adult cancer survivors: A meta-analysis. *Cancer Epidemiology, Biomarkers and Prevention, 20*(1), 123–133. doi:10.1158/1055-9965.EPI-10-0988

Dendreon Corp. (2013a). Preparing for leukapheresis and infusion days. Retrieved from http://www.provengehcp.com/PDF/Preparing%20for%20Leukapheresis%20and%20Infusion%20Day.pdf

Dendreon Corp. (2013b). Venous assessment prior to the first leukapheresis procedure for healthcare providers. Retrieved from http://www.provengehcp.com/PDF/PROF34734_Venous_Assesment_DR5_2pages.pdf

Dendreon Corp. (2014). *Provenge®* [Package insert]. Retrieved from http://www.provenge.com/pdf/prescribing-information.pdf

Drake, C.G. (2010). Prostate cancer as a model for tumour immunotherapy. *Nature Reviews Immunology, 10,* 580–593. doi:10.1038/nri2817

Kantoff, P.W., Higano, C.S., Shore, N.D., Berger, E.R., Small, E.J., Penson, D.F., ... Schellhammer, P.F. (2010). Sipuleucel-T immunotherapy for castration-resistant prostate cancer. *New England Journal of Medicine, 363,* 411–422. doi:10.1056/NEJMoa1001294

National Comprehensive Cancer Network. (2015). *NCCN Clinical Practice Guidelines in Oncology (NCCN Guidelines®): Cancer-related fatigue* [v.2.2015]. Retrieved from http://www.nccn.org/professionals/physician_gls/pdf/fatigue.pdf

Oncology Nursing Society. (2014). Putting Evidence into Practice (PEP): Fatigue. Retrieved from https://www.ons.org/practice-resources/pep/fatigue

Polovich, M., Olsen, M., & LeFebvre, K.B. (Eds.). (2014). *Chemotherapy and biotherapy guidelines and recommendations for practice* (4th ed.). Pittsburgh, PA: Oncology Nursing Society.

Vogel, W.H. (2014). Hypersensitivity reactions to antineoplastic drugs. In C.H. Yarbro, D. Wujcik, & B.H. Gobel (Eds.), *Cancer symptom management* (4th ed., pp. 115–130). Burlington, MA: Jones & Bartlett Learning.

Wenzel, J.A., Griffith, K.A., Shang, J., Thompson, C.B., Hedlin, H., Stewart, K.J., ... Mock, V. (2013). Impact of a home-based walking intervention on outcomes of sleep quality, emotional distress, and fatigue in patients undergoing treatment for solid tumors. *Oncologist, 18,* 476–484. doi:10.1634/theoncologist.2012-0278

CASE 7
Ethical Issues

Paula M. Muehlbauer, RN, MSN, AOCNS®, and Madhusree Singh, MD

A 45-year-old woman with metastatic melanoma

W.R., a 45-year-old woman, is a well-known and well-liked patient who was previously responding well to treatment for metastatic melanoma. She presents to the emergency department with blurred vision and pain and weakness in her legs. She rates her pain as 7 out of 10 on the pain scale, and her acceptable level is 4 out of 10. She is admitted to the inpatient oncology unit for further workup. It soon becomes apparent that the weakness is progressing to paralysis. This condition is nonreversible and painful, and there are no known medical interventions to slow down the progressive paralysis. The oncology team consults the palliative care team for management of her pain and other symptoms. Her pain is treated using a multimodality approach including opioids.

W.R. is alert, oriented, and of sound mind. She tells her nurse that she does not want to be placed on a ventilator and that she wants to be kept comfortable. The nurse advocates for W.R. by sharing this information with her doctors. The physicians do not talk to W.R. regarding her wishes, despite the fact that she has the ability to make her own decisions. Instead, they discuss it with her family without W.R. present.

The patient's extended family includes her husband, daughter, son, parents, two sisters, and a brother. The family is very upset and angry with the healthcare team because they thought her cancer was being cured. They hold on to the belief that there is a cure to reverse W.R.'s condition. They believe that the treatment caused this life-threatening condition. They refuse to discuss a do-not-resuscitate (DNR) order, despite her declining condition and her desire for no heroic measures.

The physicians are the main recipients of the family's anger. The physicians do not want to take away hope and are hesitant to write a DNR order. They are distressed that the therapy potentially caused her condition and are reluctant to let go. The physicians speak to the family about possible options such as a ventilator and cardiopulmonary resuscitation (CPR). The nurses are distressed over this course of action because the patient has made her wishes clear. Emotions are high, and everyone is experiencing conflict between reality, hope, and helplessness, as is common in medically futile situations (Bowers, 2006).

What is medical futility?

In this case, *futility* means that heroic measures, such as intubation and CPR, will not prevent W.R.'s death from the complications associated with her disease and treatment. Futile care is a frequent source of distress in nursing. Nurses report the most difficulty in providing quality end-of-life care because of factors that include disagreement about the dying person's care, prolongation of suffering, and physicians' reluctance to address the reality of the situation with the patient and family (Epstein & Delgado, 2010; Ferrell, 2006; Rubin, 1998; Sokol, 2009).

How can an ethics consultation assist in this case?

When conflicts arise, ethics committees, interdisciplinary team communication, collaborative practice, and institutional policies can help guide decisions. The healthcare team wants clarification of whether it is appropriate to proceed with a DNR order over the family's objections. The oncology team and palliative care team decide to consult the hospital ethics advisory team to address the conflict between the patient and family involved in the goals of care.

Figure 7-1 outlines pertinent information the hospital ethics advisory team gathers during their consultation. The team uses the Clarify, Assemble, Synthesize, Explain, and Support (CASES) approach to make recommendations (Geppart & Shelton, 2012).

Step 1: Clarify the consultation request.

The ethics consult is about the DNR decision, because the patient and family are not in agreement about healthcare decision making. W.R. feels that intubation and CPR will not add to her quality of life,

---

Figure 7-1. Information Gathered by the Ethics Team

Medical Indication
- Diagnosis: Metastatic melanoma, unresponsive to treatment
- Prognosis: Poor end-stage disease with progression to death
- Goal of treatment: Life extension versus "good death"

Patient Preferences
- Patient has capacity.
- Out-of-room decisions made by family are not consistent with patient's wishes.
- Patient does not express wishes overtly but when asked directly by nurses, she states she does not want to be intubated and feels cardiopulmonary resuscitation and intubation would be inappropriate, as her disease is progressing.

Quality of Life
- Patient has metastatic melanoma, which has progressed despite innovative treatment, and poor prognosis.
- Patient has limited mobility and is bedbound with a high level of pain.
- Patient has a loving family that is embedded in the healthcare decision making.

Contextual Features
- Family members want to continue further aggressive management, even though the patient is suffering from side effects.
- Family thinks withdrawing therapy would be "giving up."
- Palliation versus curative-invasive therapy

---

but her grieving, angry family members think not intubating means "giving up." The ethics team meets with the patient, extended family, and clinical team to discuss all the issues involved. They clarify their role as a consulting service that can improve the quality of decision making, but that, ultimately, the decision will be made with clinicians and W.R., who has capacity to make her own decisions.

Step 2: Assemble the relevant information.

The team gathers information from all sources, including the patient, family, nurses, and other treating clinicians. The overarching concern is whether ignoring the patient's wishes not to undergo CPR and intubation is the right thing to do. Issues of nonbeneficial treatment are also considered, as W.R.'s metastatic melanoma is no longer responding to her chemotherapy.

Step 3: Synthesize the information.

The team calls a family meeting, where all the treating clinicians, nurses, and family members have an opportunity to share their perspectives. The ethical principle of patient autonomy is discussed.

Because W.R. has capacity, she should be able to make an informed decision related to her health care.

Step 4: Explain the synthesis.

The ethics team speaks with the clinical team, family members, and W.R. to share the results of its deliberation. The team puts a note in W.R.'s chart explaining the decision-making process.

Step 5: Support the consultation process.

The ethics team remains available for follow-up to questions and concerns from the clinical team.

Key Points

- Establish and discuss goals of care with both patient and family present.
- Discuss benefits versus risks of therapy with patient and family.
- Conduct an ethics consultation using the CASES approach.

Nurses act as patient advocates and liaisons between patients, family members, and providers. Nurses often address issues such as religious beliefs, intrafamily issues, grief, guilt, distrust, value differences, and secondary gains (Prince-Paul & Daly, 2010). With the help of the ethics team, W.R. and her family have an opportunity to clarify her diagnosis and prognosis, share information in plain language rather than medical lingo, and discuss what it means to "do everything."

Conclusion

After the ethics team consults, the healthcare team and palliative care team collaborate with the family and eventually agree to honor W.R.'s wishes. Her code status is changed to DNR. She dies comfortably several days later with her family at her bedside.

After W.R.'s death, a member of the palliative care team meets with the nurses to debrief. They express their discomfort over the entire situation and talk about plans for future patient care concerns. Moral distress occurs in medically futile situations when advocacy for the patient or family is not successful or when hope is unrealistic. Moral distress causes psychological pain and imbalance when nurses perceive they are in a situation where they are unable to do the right thing (Gallagher, 2010; McCue, 2010). The ethics team acknowledges the distress the nurses feel and provides them with an approach to address future morally distressing situations (American Association of Critical-Care Nurses, 2004; McCue, 2010) (see Table 7-1).

Table 7-1. Four A's of Handling Moral Distress

Step	Description	Goal
Ask	Review the symptoms of moral distress and ask, "Is this what I am feeling? Are others feeling or acting the same way?"	To be aware that moral distress is present
Affirm	Determine what part of moral integrity is being threatened, and validate these perceptions with others. What can or should be done to address this feeling?	To make a commitment to deal with the distress and affirm professional obligation as a nurse
Assess	Combine the facts and identify the sources of distress.	To assess readiness to make an action plan
Act	Create a plan and initiate strategies to make the desired changes. Consider the pros and cons of each action and know what drawbacks await.	By acting, the nurse preserves one's individual integrity.

Note. Based on information from American Association of Critical-Care Nurses, 2004; McCue, 2010.

References

American Association of Critical-Care Nurses. (2004). The 4A's to rise above moral distress. Retrieved from http://www.aacn.org/WD/Practice/Docs/4As_to_Rise_Above_Moral_Distress.pdf

Bowers, L. (2006). Ethical issues along the cancer continuum. In R.M. Carroll-Johnson, L.M. Gorman, & N.J. Bush (Eds.), *Psychosocial nursing care along the cancer continuum* (2nd ed., pp. 551–564). Pittsburgh, PA: Oncology Nursing Society.

Epstein, E.G., & Delgado, S. (2010). Understanding and addressing moral distress. *Online Journal of Issues in Nursing, 15*(3), Manuscript 1. doi:10.3912/OJIN.Vol15No03Man01

Ferrell, B. (2006). Understanding the moral distress of nurses witnessing medically futile care. *Oncology Nursing Forum, 33*, 922–930. doi:10.1188/06.ONF.922-930

Gallagher, A. (2010). Moral distress and moral courage in everyday nursing practice. *Online Journal of Issues in Nursing, 16*(2). doi:10.3912/OJIN.Vol16No02PPT03

Geppart, C.M.A., & Shelton, W.N. (2012). A comparison of general medical and clinical ethics consultations: What can we learn from each other? *Mayo Clinic Proceedings, 87*, 381–389. doi:10.1016/j.mayocp.2011.10.010

McCue, C. (2010). Using the AACN framework to alleviate moral distress. *Online Journal of Issues in Nursing, 16*(1). doi:10.3912/OJIN.Vol16No01PPT02

Prince-Paul, M., & Daly, B.J. (2010). Ethical considerations in palliative care. In B.R. Ferrell & N. Coyle (Eds.), *Oxford textbook of palliative nursing* (3rd ed., pp. 1157–1171). New York, NY: Oxford University Press.

Rubin, S.B. (1998). *When doctors say no: The battleground of medical futility.* Bloomington, IN: Indiana University Press.

Sokol, D.K. (2009). The slipperiness of futility. *BMJ, 338,* b2222. doi:10.1136/bmj .b2222

CASE 8
Chemotherapy Safety

Michael Smart, RN, BSN, OCN®

A 35-year-old man with colon cancer

P.B. is a 35-year-old divorced father of three children. He works in food service, generally eats a high-fat diet, smokes cigarettes, and drinks alcoholic beverages on a daily basis. He experiences abdominal pain, which he attributes to constipation. The pain becomes progressively worse over a two-week period, and he begins having severe nausea and vomiting. During an emergency department visit, P.B. is told he likely has a viral infection and is sent home with a prescription for ondansetron for nausea and dicyclomine for abdominal cramping.

P.B.'s symptoms subside over the next few days. Two weeks later, he experiences more severe sharp abdominal pain with nausea and vomiting, and he returns to the emergency department. This time, he is admitted with a bowel obstruction that requires surgery.

During surgery, a 12 in. (30.5 cm) tumor originating in the cecum (proximal colon) is found. Debulking of the tumor requires resecting the colon and placing an ileostomy. Pathology confirms a diagnosis of adenocarcinoma. P.B. is referred to an oncologist, who reviews the pathology prior to talking about treatment options, such as chemotherapy, with P.B.

Why is confirming the pathology important in deciding the course of chemotherapy?

Chemotherapy is not a "one-size-fits-all" treatment for cancer. Pathology helps determine which regimen is likely to be most beneficial. Pathologic confirmation should be documented in the patient record (Neuss et al., 2013). After discussing P.B.'s treatment options, the oncologist develops a plan to proceed with the chemotherapy regimen FOLFOX6 14 days after the removal of P.B.'s abdominal incision staples.

FOLFOX6 entails administration of folinic acid (commonly known as leucovorin), fluorouracil (5-FU), and oxaliplatin.

P.B. asks, "Why do I have colon cancer? I thought smoking was supposed to give you lung cancer."

Smoking, high-cholesterol diet, and regular consumption of alcohol are all risk factors associated with increased colorectal cancer occurrence (López, Albero, & Rodríguez-Montes, 2014). Even so, colorectal cancer is typically a disease of older adults, and screening is usually not recommended until age 50 for patients at average risk for developing colorectal cancer (American Cancer Society, 2015).

P.B.'s young age at diagnosis is unusual and points to the importance of considering inherited traits that might predispose other family members to colon cancer (Stigliano, Sanchez-Mete, Martayan, & Anti, 2014). Family history reveals an uncle who had colon cancer in his thirties. The oncologist recommends that other first-degree relatives, including P.B.'s children, begin colon screening at age 25 (10 years younger than the age at which P.B. has been diagnosed).

"If this is so serious, why am I not starting chemotherapy right away?"

P.B. asks his nurse this question when he is being discharged from the hospital. What might be an appropriate answer?

The planned chemotherapy will suppress his immune system and possibly delay healing of his surgical wound. It was important to allow time for healing to avoid complications such as wound infections. This is balanced with the risks of delaying chemotherapy postoperatively; too long of a delay can result in less than optimal outcomes (Yoshida et al., 2011). The plan is to start chemotherapy as soon as is reasonably safe to do so.

The treatment regimen, FOLFOX6, consists of chemotherapy in two-week cycles over a six-month period. One week before chemotherapy starts, P.B. meets with an oncology nurse to review his plan of care. Ensuring the patient's understanding of the treatment and anticipated side effects before initiation of therapy is an important safety standard and should be documented in the patient record

(Neuss et al., 2013). P.B. is also provided with written information regarding his chemotherapy regimen to review at home.

Why is it best practice to do chemotherapy teaching ahead of time?

Allowing time before initiation of chemotherapy enables the patient to process information, become an informed participant in care, and possibly better manage anticipated side effects (Yesilbalkan, Karadakovan, & Göker, 2009).

On treatment day, P.B. goes to his oncologist's clinic for chemotherapy. The RN assigned to P.B. verifies that the physician orders for the day are consistent with the documented plan for FOLFOX6. The facility maintains copies of the most commonly used chemotherapy regimens, including FOLFOX6, for nurses to reference. There is a policy stating that any deviations from standard regimens require documentation of the rationale in the medical record. This is consistent with the American Society of Clinical Oncology and Oncology Nursing Society chemotherapy administration safety standards (Neuss et al., 2013).

The RN notes that there are no changes from standard FOLFOX6 in P.B.'s orders. In addition to premedications, the chemotherapy orders consist of

- Oxaliplatin 100 mg/m² and leucovorin 400 mg/m² IV over two hours
- 5-FU 400 mg/m² IV bolus
- 5-FU 3,000 mg/m² IV by continuous infusion over 46 hours.

While establishing P.B.'s IV access via an implantable port placed during his hospitalization, the RN reviews the prior teaching about chemotherapy to ensure P.B. understands the potential complications and side effects of chemotherapy.

What unique precautions related to oxaliplatin does P.B. need to know?

Exposure to cold can cause very painful sensations following oxaliplatin therapy. P.B. is encouraged to avoid cold during the days following chemotherapy. Resolution of this side effect usually occurs within five days following therapy but may last longer (Sanofi-Aventis, 2014). It is important for the nurse to cover not only common chemotherapy side effects, such as myelosuppression, but also the unique side effects related to the specific drugs patients receive.

The oncology nurse talks to P.B. about why she wears personal protective equipment (PPE), including chemotherapy gown and chemotherapy gloves, while administering chemotherapy.

Why is wearing personal protective equipment important for nurses when administering chemotherapy?

Cytotoxic chemotherapy agents are hazardous drugs. Exposure to the agents by healthcare providers can have acute side effects similar to patients' experiences (e.g., nausea, hair loss). Exposures can also result in serious long-term consequences such as increased risk of cancer (Polovich, 2011). The nurse emphasizes her daily handling of chemotherapy and therefore the need to minimize her personal exposure. She explains that the benefits of chemotherapy outweigh the risks for patients receiving treatment for cancer but would pose only a risk for staff.

What are the guidelines for the use of personal protective equipment for chemotherapy administration, and what additional precautions are recommended?

Chemotherapy gowns are single-use gowns. They should be made from material that is resistant to chemical permeation and have a closed front (i.e., tied in the back, not buttoned up the front). Nurses should wear double chemotherapy gloves when handling chemotherapy. The inner gloves are donned before the gown, and the second pair is applied over the gown cuff (Polovich, 2011). PPE should be removed carefully and discarded after use to prevent transfer of contamination. Deficits in nursing knowledge and failure of employers to provide appropriate PPE have been cited as reasons for nurses not following National Institute of Occupational Safety and Health guidelines when handling hazardous drugs (Polovich & Martin, 2011).

P.B.'s chemotherapy is transported from the pharmacy in a sealed zipper-lock bag. Before removing the chemotherapy from the bag for verification at the chairside, the nurse visually confirms that the chemotherapy is not leaking and that two clamps are on the IV tubing to prevent leakage, which is in accordance with the clinic policy.

Closed system transfer devices (CSTDs) are sometimes used to prevent leakage from IV tubing in case the clamps loosen. For drug administration, a CSTD prevents fluid from escaping the IV tubing until it is attached to a Luer-lock IV connection or companion CSTD on the patient's IV. CSTDs reduce healthcare workers' exposure to hazardous drugs (Polovich, 2011).

What steps are recommended for promoting patient safety related to chemotherapy?

P.B.'s nurse has another chemotherapy-competent RN verify the chemotherapy and documents that this verification occurred. They verify P.B.'s identity using two identifiers, name and date of birth. The correct drug, dose, route, volume, and rate of administration are checked, as well as the physical integrity of the drugs (e.g., precipitate formation). When chemotherapy is prepared ahead of time, the expiration date and time are also checked (Neuss et al., 2013).

P.B. receives his oxaliplatin, leucovorin, and bolus 5-FU without experiencing any infusion reactions or side effects. He is sent home with the continuous infusion of 5-FU after two nurses verify the correct portable pump programming. Discharge instructions include a review of expected side effects, an appointment to return on day 3 to have the pump disconnected, and suggestions regarding how to bathe without contaminating his IV site.

On day 4, P.B. experienced mouth sores. He found these to be very painful, but they did not interfere with his ability to eat and drink. He was not overly concerned, as he had been forewarned to expect this side effect. He used saline rinses after eating to keep his oral cavity clean as suggested by the nurse, and the sores resolved before his second cycle of FOLFOX6.

Which chemotherapy agent was most likely responsible for the mouth sores (oral mucositis or stomatitis)?

5-FU is commonly associated with oral mucositis (Polovich, Olsen, & LeFebvre, 2014). During his second cycle, P.B. said he heard that chewing on ice during chemotherapy could prevent the oral sores. The nurse explains that chewing on ice during bolus 5-FU can reduce the severity of oral mucositis, but the need for cold precautions because of the oxaliplatin is a contraindication for this measure (Polovich et al., 2014; Sanofi-Aventis, 2014).

During his visit for cycle 2, P.B. shares his experience with cold sensitivity after his first treatment. He had just been thinking how happy he was to not experience nausea, when he reached into his refrigerator to get something to eat. He experienced an immediate and severe burning "electrical" sensation that served as a dramatic reminder to avoid cold. After two days, he tried a milkshake but experienced excruciating pain on swallowing. On the fourth day, he decided to test his cold tolerance by grabbing an ice cube out of the freezer and squeezing it in his hand. Unfortunately, he discovered that four days was still too soon.

The nurse explains that neurologic toxicities can vary from one patient to the next. The nurse suggests that a good rule of thumb is to avoid cold exposure for at least four to five days, and, when stopping cold precautions, to go slowly. For example, try a cool drink instead of an ice-cold one.

As subsequent cycles do not bring him any surprises, P.B. continues to stay on therapy as initially planned. He shares his experiences with his nurses. He also suggests other measures he "learned along the way," such as wearing slippers around the house, because even the cold tiles of the bathroom floor were bothersome. The nurse assures him that this information will be incorporated in teaching for other patients.

Key Points

Nurses are responsible for protecting both patients and themselves:
- Ensure that the regimen is appropriate for disease.
- Independently verify dose calculations.
- Confirm that medications delivered match what is ordered.
- Educate patients about side effects and potential consequences.
- Wear two pairs of chemotherapy gloves and a fluid-resistant, single-use chemotherapy gown.
- Appropriately handle and discard chemotherapy waste.

Conclusion

Chemotherapy agents are an important weapon in the fight against cancer, but they do not come without risk. Patients can be prepared through education about known side effects and potential consequences. Nurses and other healthcare providers who handle these agents are also at risk for health consequences related to unintended exposure. Reducing exposure risk can be accomplished through appropriate handling of the agents as well as use of PPE.

References

American Cancer Society. (2015). American Cancer Society recommendations for colorectal cancer early detection. Retrieved from http://www.cancer.org/cancer/colonandrectumcancer/moreinformation/colonandrectumcancerearly detection/colorectal-cancer-early-detection-acs-recommendations

López, P.J., Albero, J.S., & Rodríguez-Montes, J.A. (2014). Primary and secondary prevention of colorectal cancer. *Clinical Medicine Insights: Gastroenterology, 7*, 33–46. doi:10.4137/CGast.S14039

Neuss, M.N., Polovich, M., McNiff, K., Esper, P., Gilmore, T.R., LeFebvre, K.B., & Jacobson, J.O. (2013). 2013 updated American Society of Clinical Oncology/Oncology Nursing Society chemotherapy administration safety standards including standards for the safe administration and management of oral chemotherapy. *Oncology Nursing Forum, 40*, 225–233. doi:10.1188/13.ONF.40-03AP2

Polovich, M. (Ed.). (2011). *Safe handling of hazardous drugs* (2nd ed.). Pittsburgh, PA: Oncology Nursing Society.

Polovich, M., & Martin, S. (2011). Nurses' use of hazardous drug-handling precautions and awareness of national safety guidelines. *Oncology Nursing Forum, 38*, 718–726. doi:10.1188/11.ONF.718-726

Polovich, M., Olsen, M., & LeFebvre, K.B. (Eds.). (2014). *Chemotherapy and biotherapy guidelines and recommendations for practice* (4th ed.). Pittsburgh, PA: Oncology Nursing Society.

Sanofi-Aventis. (2014). *Eloxatin® (oxaliplatin)* [Package insert]. Bridgewater, NJ: Author.

Stigliano, V., Sanchez-Mete, L., Martayan, A., & Anti, M. (2014). Early-onset colorectal cancer: A sporadic or inherited disease. *World Journal of Gastroenterology, 20*, 12420–12430. doi:10.3748/wjg.v20.i35.12420

Yesilbalkan, Ö.U., Karadakovan, A., & Göker, E. (2009). The effectiveness of nursing education as an intervention to decrease fatigue in Turkish patients receiving chemotherapy [Online exclusive]. *Oncology Nursing Forum, 36*, E215–E222. doi:10.1188/09.ONF.E215-E222

Yoshida, Y., Hoshina, S., Shiwaku, H., Beppu, R., Tanimura, S., Tanaka, S., & Yamashita, Y. (2011). Early start of chemotherapy after resection of primary colon cancer with synchronous multiple liver metastases: A case report. *Case Reports in Oncology, 4*, 250–254. doi:10.1159/000328805

CASE 9
Oral Chemotherapy

Patricia Jakel, RN, MN, AOCN®

A 16-year-old girl with chronic myeloid leukemia

A.L. is 16 years old when she presents with easy bruising and extreme fatigue after walking two blocks from high school. She has splenomegaly 2 cm below the left costal margin during her first visit to a children's hospital. Her complete blood count reveals the following: white blood cell (WBC) count of 299,000/mm³, hemoglobin of 11.4 g/dl, and platelet count of 305,000/mm³. Bone marrow biopsy shows 1% blasts, 13% promyelocytes, 24% myelocytes, 15% metamyelocytes, 16% bands, 15% segmented neutrophils, 7% eosinophils, and 1% basophils. Fluorescence in situ hybridization for molecular cytogenetic analysis reveals the presence of the Philadelphia chromosome in all 20 metaphases, confirming the diagnosis of chronic myeloid leukemia (CML) or chronic myelongenous leukemia, chronic phase (see Table 9-1). A.L. is living in foster care with four other foster siblings with ages ranging from 4 to 16 years old. Her foster mother is with her at the time of diagnosis.

What are the key statistics about chronic myeloid leukemia?

CML is a disease of older adults, with a median age of 65; however, a growing number of younger patients are being diagnosed. The median age in the clinical trials for CML has declined by at least 10 years, according to a recent publication (Pemmaraju & Cortes, 2014).

A.L. is started on imatinib 400 mg/day, resulting in normalization of her WBC count within eight weeks (see Table 9-2 for CML treatment). The nurse practitioner (NP) provides extensive educa-

Table 9-1. Phases of Chronic Myeloid Leukemia

Phase	Common Presenting Signs	Chromosomal Abnormalities	White Blood Cell Count	Blasts	Other
Chronic phase	None or possible nonspecific symptoms, including fatigue, weight loss, fevers, night sweats, stomach pain, or fullness	Philadelphia chromosome and the *BCR-ABL* genetic mutation	Elevated: 50,000–5,000,000/mm^3 or higher; controlled with treatment	< 15%	Platelets elevated Basophils elevated Control with treatment Spleen likely enlarged
Accelerated phase	Loss of control of blood counts	Possible additional chromosomal abnormalities and genetic mutations	Abnormal	15%–30%	Abnormal platelets Basophils > 20% Spleen likely enlarged
Blast crisis	Bruising, internal bleeding, infections	Possible additional chromosomal abnormalities and genetic mutations	Abnormal	< 30%	Abnormal platelets Basophils > 20% Spleen likely enlarged

Note. Based on information from Negrin & Schiffer, 2014.

Table 9-4. Common Reasons for Nonadherence to Oral Anticancer Drugs *(Continued)*	
Reason for Nonadherence	**Interventions**
Functional difficulties	• Use of pill bottles with easy-open caps, but educate patient about keeping the medication away from pets and children • Support from family, friends, or healthcare provider in the home
High cost of drugs	• Person in the practice working with the patient and insurance • Pharmaceutical financial assistance • Organizations and advocacy groups
Inadequate follow-up	• Assess if patient's family and friends can support and drive patient • Call patient between appointments

Lack of confidence in the treatment	• Support groups (in person and online)
	• Online support, including but not limited to
	  – www.curetoday.com
	  – www.cancercare.org
	  – www.mylifeline.org

Note. Based on information from Dalby et al., 2013; Hartigan, 2003; Winkeljohn, 2010.	

ogy nurses, which provides resources, tools, and interviewing techniques to improve adherence.

What other issues are associated with appropriate dosing of oral chemotherapy?

Overadherence is also an important nursing concern with the use of oral chemotherapy (Spoelstra et al., 2013). Overadherence is described as taking extra doses of oral chemotherapy on a single day, during rest periods, during drug-free days, or after the drug cycle was completed. The authors reported that patients started taking the oral medications immediately upon receipt from the pharmacy, including medications received by mail, while acknowledging that they had yet to understand the treatment plan. Nurses need to help patients and families understand, and nurses need to monitor the oral chemotherapy regimen.

A.L. is being treated at a children's hospital, is in foster care, and has run away on numerous occasions. She is nonadherent with her oral chemotherapy, which contributes to the loss of cytogenetic response after a year and a half on an oral tyrosine kinase inhibitor.

Key Point

- In a patient with CML, adherence to treatment is the most important factor in determining molecular response (Marin et al., 2010).

Two years after being diagnosed with CML, A.L.'s bone marrow aspirate shows 20% of the marrow metaphases have the Philadelphia chromosome. Because of a lack of the cytogenetic response, she is switched to dasatinib 100 mg/day (see Table 9-2). A.L. presents to the hematology clinic located at a large academic medical center. A.L. states she is dissatisfied with her care at the children's hospital and is seeking a second opinion. The NP completes a careful assessment, but it is still unclear if A.L. adhered to the medication schedule of the dasatinib, and there is no recent documentation of assessment of her disease.

What are the safety considerations for patients taking oral chemotherapy?

Ensuring patient safety during administration of oral chemotherapy presents healthcare providers, patients, and families with many unique challenges. ONS and ASCO recommend that assessment of patients on oral chemotherapy should include socioeconomic, psychosocial, and financial aspects, in addition to determination of their ability to administer the medication in a safe and consistent manner (Neuss et al., 2013). A.L. started her oral chemotherapy living in foster care with other young children. In that setting, it would be easy to identify many potential risks to her and others around her.

What are the safety considerations for home care?

Nurses should assess and educate patients and their caregivers on safe storage, administration, disposal, and cleaning of any contaminated materials, including pill containers, counters, and any contact surfaces. The materials can be cleaned with soap and water (Polovich, Olsen, & LeFebvre, 2014). Patients and their caregivers need to be assessed as to whether they are unable to open a child safety cap, instructed to keep all oral chemotherapy agents in their original containers, and reminded not to keep expired medications (Goodin et al., 2011).

Oral chemotherapy agents can remain in the gut for five to seven days, so patients' stool will contain by-products of the anticancer agents (Griffin, 2003). Patient education needs to include that the patient should use a separate bathroom if possible, double flush the toilet with the lid down, wash the patient's clothes and bedding separately if soiled with body fluids or chemotherapy, and minimize the number of people handling patient waste. Anyone handling the medication, waste, or chemotherapy-soiled materials must wear gloves (Polovich et al., 2014). Items contaminated with anticancer medications should not be put in regular trash. Patients should receive a hard plastic chemotherapy waste container obtained by the homecare company if required for safe disposal of the medication. A chemotherapy waste container should also be used when anticancer medications are given in skilled nursing/assisted living facilities and in hospitals with non-oncology units. Figure 9-1 lists specific recommendations on safe handling of oral chemotherapy agents for patients and their caregivers.

Key Points

- Imatinib is listed as a hazardous drug by the National Institute for Occupational Safety and Health (NIOSH) (2014).
- When people other than the patient handle oral hazardous drugs, they should do so wearing personal protective equipment.
- If oral anticancer agents need to be crushed, cut, opened, or dissolved, trained personnel must use a biologic safety cabinet for these tasks (Neuss et al., 2013).

A.L. leaves foster care at the age of 18 and moves in with her half-sister. She is immediately referred to social work to assist with medication adherence. On her first visit to the clinic, it becomes

Figure 9-1. Specific Recommendations for Patients and Caregivers: Dos and Don'ts

Dos for Oral Chemotherapy
- On receiving your prescription, review the package label, specifically checking medication name and dosage.
- Ensure that you completely understand when and how to take the medication and ask questions if there is any confusion.
- Transport and store medicine as instructed and as outlined in the packaging label.
- Use gloves, if possible, and wash hands thoroughly before and after glove application.* If gloves are not worn, tip tablets and capsules from their container/blister pack directly into a disposable medicine cup.
- Administer the medication as instructed.
- Keep a journal of adverse effects. Make a list of adverse effects for which the healthcare professional needs to be contacted immediately.
- Consider using adherence devices. Use separate devices for cytotoxic and noncytotoxic agents.
- Report any overdosing immediately.
- Keep information ready for necessary action in the event of accidental exposure (including emesis and accidental ingestion).
- Return wet, damaged, unused, discontinued, or expired medications to the pharmacist or hospital for disposal.
- Report all medications (prescription and nonprescription as well as complementary and alternative medicines) and any specific dietary requirements to the healthcare provider/prescriber at the time of assessment and consultation. Inform other healthcare professionals (e.g., surgeons and dentists) that you are on oral chemotherapy.
- Minimize the number of individuals coming in contact with the cytotoxic medications.
- Wash the patient's clothes and bed linen separately from other items.
- Double-flush the toilet after use, during use of, and 4 to 7 days after discontinuing oral chemotherapy.

Don'ts for Oral Chemotherapy
- Double-up on doses, unless instructed by a healthcare professional.
- Leave medication in open areas, near sources of water, under direct sunlight, or where they can be accessed by children or pets.
- Crush, break, or chew tablets.
- Share prescriptions or medication.
- Store medications in the areas where food or drinks are stored or consumed.
- Assume that oral chemotherapy is safer than intravenous chemotherapy.
- Skip doses unless instructed by your physician.
- Discard medication down the toilet or in the garbage.

---

* It is recommended that caregivers wear gloves at all times while handling oral chemotherapeutic agents as well as contaminated items in order to minimize risk of exposure.

Note. From "Safe Handling of Oral Chemotherapeutic Agents in Clinical Practice: Recommendations From an International Pharmacy Panel," by S. Goodin, N. Griffith, B. Chen, K. Chuk, M. Dauphars, C. Doreau, ... K. Meier, 2011, *Journal of Oncology Practice, 7,* p. 10. Copyright 2011 by American Society of Clinical Oncology. Reprinted with permission.

clear that her ability to follow transplant requirements for an unrelated transplant with very little family support is doubtful. A.L.'s case is presented at the bone marrow transplant conference, and an intense social work assessment is completed.

After a careful assessment at the clinic, the patient is changed to ponatinib 100 mg/day with a follow-up visit the next day with the NP to review the medication. Initial education is completed, and the prescription is filled at the hospital outpatient pharmacy to ensure drug supply. A.L. does not return to the clinic for two weeks, missing two appointments, but her complete blood count is starting to normalize, so it appears she is taking the medication appropriately.

What are the potential medication errors related to oral chemotherapy?

Prescribing oral chemotherapy has many unique challenges and opportunities. The 2013 standards from ASCO and ONS (Neuss et al., 2013) describe the requirements for oral chemotherapy prescriptions: two identifiers, drug name, date, method of dose calculation including body surface area if applicable, quantity, dose (rounded to the nearest tablet size, no trailing zeros), route, frequency, duration of treatment days, number of refills, and a time limit of the prescription to ensure that the patient returns for an evaluation.

Prescribers should provide the information listed above to any pharmacy dispensing oral chemotherapy agents. When these prescriptions are filled by pharmacies without much experience with oral anticancer agents, patients must assume a greater responsibility for verifying and ensuring that they are taking the right dose at the right time. Some issues identified in retail pharmacies include stocking of medications, insurance problems, unclear label instructions, and lack of knowledge by retail pharmacists (Simchowitz et al., 2010). The use of mail-order pharmacies is increasingly common and is not without problems. Manufacturers and distributors should package these medications to avoid contamination, use durable packaging, label the drugs as hazardous, and make them tamper proof (Goodin et al., 2011).

Table 9-5 contains recommendations for verification of oral chemotherapy doses in various home settings (Griffin, 2003). This is a useful guide for nurses in educating patients and families about dual verification in settings outside the clinics and hospitals.

Table 9-5. Safety Guidelines for Administration of Oral Agents in Various Settings	
Setting	Recommendations
Patient's home: Important to encourage a double-check process within the home	• Patient and family member • Two family members • Patient and friend • Family member and friend • Two friends
Assisted living center: Registered nurses or licensed vocation nurses often not available, depending on the laws of individual states	• Two nurses (if available) • Nurse and medication technician • Nurse and other staff member • Nurse and patient • Medication technician and patient
Nursing home or hospital with no oncology nurse	• Two nurses
Hospital with oncology services	• Two oncology nurses • Two nurses who have completed the Oncology Nursing Society Oral Therapies for Cancer Course
Note. Based on information from Griffin, 2003.	

A.L.'s half-sister and aunt agree to be her primary support for an unrelated transplant. A.L. is not open to allowing others to help and does not adhere to the family's rules for her safety, such as not staying out all night, taking her oral anticancer agents on time, and reporting for her follow-up appointments as required. Unfortunately, she is admitted to the hospital in blast crisis and dies within several days.

Conclusion

This is an unfortunate case where the lack of adherence played a major role in this patient's demise from CML. Oral chemotherapy agents allow for flexibility, patient control, multiple treatment choices, and improved quality of life with less travel and more time away from clinics, but many challenges also arise. The multiple risks associated with oral chemotherapy agents include medication error, potential exposure to patients and others, and overall compromised patient safety. Osterberg and Blaschke (2005) suggested that medication adherence can be improved by patient education, improved dosing schedule, increased clinic hours, and improved communication between healthcare providers and patients. Nurses are positioned to address many issues with patients receiving oral anticancer agents. Oral agents can work well, but only if patients take the medication correctly and maintain safe care. Sadly, A.L. could not follow the treatment plan despite many interventions by healthcare workers and those who cared for her.

References

Dalby, C.K., Nesbitt, M., Frechette, C.A., Kennerley, K., Lacoursiere, L.H., & Buswell, L. (2013). Standardization of initial chemotherapy teaching to improve care. *Clinical Journal of Oncology Nursing, 17,* 472–475.

Goodin, S., Griffith, N., Chen, B., Chuk, K., Daouphars, M., Doreau, C., ... Meier, K. (2011). Safe handling of oral chemotherapeutic agents in clinical practice: Recommendations from an international pharmacy panel. *Journal of Oncology Practice, 7,* 7–12. doi:10.1200/JOP.2010.000068

Griffin, E. (2003). Safety considerations and safe handling of oral chemotherapy agents. *Clinical Journal of Oncology Nursing, 7*(Suppl. 6), 25–29. doi:10.1188/03 .CJON.S6.25-29

Halfdanarson, T.R., & Jatoi, A. (2010). Oral cancer chemotherapy: The critical interplay between patient education and patient safety. *Current Oncology Reports, 12,* 247–252. doi:10.1007/s11912-010-0103-6

Hartigan, K. (2003). Patient education: The cornerstone of successful oral chemotherapy treatment. *Clinical Journal of Oncology Nursing, 7,* 21–24. doi:10.1188/03 .CJON.S6.21-24

Mancini, R., McBride, A., & Kruczynski, M. (2013). Oral oncolytics: Part 1—Financial, adherence, and management challenges. *Oncology, 27,* 742–744.

Marin, D., Bazeos, A., Mahon, F.X., Eliasson, L., Milojkovic, D., Bua, M., ... Khorashad, J.S. (2010). Adherence is the critical factor for achieving molecular responses in patients with chronic myeloid leukemia who achieve complete cytogenetic responses on imatinib. *Journal of Clinical Oncology, 28,* 2381–2388. doi:10.1200/JCO.2009.26.3087

National Comprehensive Cancer Network. (2015). *NCCN Clinical Practice Guidelines in Oncology (NCCN Guidelines®): Chronic myelogenous leukemia* [v.1.2015]. Retrieved from http://www.nccn.org/professionals/physician_gls/pdf/cml.pdf

National Institute for Occupational Safety and Health. (2014). NIOSH list of antineoplastic and other hazardous drugs in healthcare settings, 2014. Retrieved from http://www.cdc.gov/niosh/docs/2014-138/pdfs/2014-138.pdf

Negrin, R.S., & Schiffer, C.A. (2014). Clinical use of tyrosine kinase inhibitors for chronic myeloid leukemia [UpToDate]. Retrieved from http://www.uptodate. com/contents/clinical-use-of-tyrosine-kinase-inhibitors-for-chronic-myeloid -leukemia

Neuss, M.N., Polovich, M., McNiff, K., Esper, P., Gilmore, T.R., LeFebvre, K.B., & Jacobson, J.O. (2013). 2013 updated American Society of Clinical Oncology/Oncology Nursing Society chemotherapy administration safety standards including standards for the safe administration and management of oral chemotherapy. *Oncology Nursing Forum, 40*, 225–233. doi:10.1188/13.ONF.40-03AP2

Oncology Nursing Society. (2009). *Tools for oral adherence toolkit.* Retrieved from https://www.ons.org/sites/default/files/oral%20adherence%20toolkit.pdf

Osterberg, L., & Blaschke, T. (2005). Adherence to medication. *New England Journal of Medicine, 353*, 487–497. doi:10.1056/NEJMra050100

Pemmaraju, N., & Cortes, J. (2014). Chronic myeloid leukemia in adolescents and young adults: Patient characteristics, outcomes and review of the literature. *Acta Haematologica, 132*, 298–306. doi:10.1159/000363434

Polovich, M., Olsen, M., & LeFebvre, K.B. (Eds.). (2014). *Chemotherapy and biotherapy guidelines and recommendations for practice* (4th ed.). Pittsburgh, PA: Oncology Nursing Society.

Roop, J.C., & Wu, H.-S. (2014). Current practice patterns for oral chemotherapy: Results of a national survey. *Oncology Nursing Forum, 41*, 185–194. doi:10.1188/14.ONF.41-02AP

Simchowitz, B., Shiman, L., Spencer, J., Brouillard, D., Gross, A., Connor, M., & Weingart, S.N. (2010). Perceptions and experiences of patients receiving oral chemotherapy. *Clinical Journal of Oncology Nursing, 14*, 447–453. doi:10.1188/10.CJON.447-453

Spoelstra, S.L., Given, B.A., Given, C.W., Grant, M., Sikorskii, A., You, M., & Decker, V. (2013). Issues related to overadherence to oral chemotherapy or targeted agents. *Clinical Journal of Oncology Nursing, 17*, 604–609. doi:10.1188/13.CJON.17-06AP

Winkeljohn, D. (2010). Adherence to oral cancer therapies: Nursing interventions. *Clinical Journal of Oncology Nursing, 14*, 461–466. doi:10.1188/10.CJON.461-466

Yagasaki, K., & Komatsu, H. (2013). The need for a nursing presence in oral chemotherapy. *Clinical Journal of Oncology Nursing, 17*, 512–516. doi:10.1188/13.CJON.512-516

CASE 10
Vascular Access

Patrice E. Roberts, RN, BSN, OCN®, and MiKaela Olsen, MS, APRN-CNS, AOCNS®

A 58-year-old man with inflammatory myofibroblastic sarcoma

J.G. is a 58-year-old man who presents with a rapidly enlarging mass in the first intertriginous space of his right hand. The mass is painful and limits mobility of his index finger. Pathology from an incisional biopsy reveals a low-grade fibroinflammatory sarcoma. Computed tomography (CT) scans and other metastatic workup are negative. Although discussed, he does not want to proceed with an amputation. J.G. undergoes a radical resection of a low-grade soft tissue sarcoma of the right hand with reconstruction.

At his six-month follow-up appointment, a magnetic resonance imaging scan shows J.G. has a recurrent mass encasing and infiltrating the flexor digitorum profundus of the right finger. The mass abuts the flexor digitorum superficialis of the right finger and the flexor tendons of the small fingers. Repeat CT scans of the chest, abdomen, and pelvis are performed, and he is noted to have multiple diffuse bilateral pulmonary nodules, suspicious for metastasis. The medical oncologist advises systemic chemotherapy. J.G. is recommended to receive MAI chemotherapy, which includes mesna, doxorubicin (Adriamycin®), and ifosfamide. J.G. needs a central venous access device (CVAD) in order to receive this therapy. Prior to line placement, J.G. will meet with the treatment team to discuss his options and help choose the device best suited for his lifestyle. Several factors will be taken into account when determining which CVAD will be the best option for the patient. This will be discussed in the next section.

What should the nurse ask the patient in order to adequately assess what type of venous access is appropriate?

To choose the most appropriate venous access, a thorough assessment should be performed. The assessment should include patient preference and treatment-specific requirements. How does J.G. feel about a central line placed in his chest versus his arm? What existing activity limitations does J.G. have, and what does he want to be able to continue to do? What kind of job does J.G. have, and does he have a caregiver who can help him with his line care? Does J.G. have the resources to obtain central line maintenance supplies, or will he need to find transportation to come to a facility for his line care?

In order for J.G. to make an informed decision, he will need education on the various catheter types that are appropriate for his situation. The provider should assess his understanding of each catheter and the risks and benefits prior to obtaining consent for the insertion. Another important question is whether he will need frequent CT scans for evaluation of his disease.

J.G. will be receiving doxorubicin, which is a vesicant chemotherapy drug. *Vesicants* are drugs or agents that are capable of causing tissue necrosis if extravasated (Elsevier Mosby, 2012). J.G. expresses concern about his existing limitations with his right hand and is worried about the number of venipunctures he has already received in his left hand and arm. "I need to be able to use my left hand for everything," he explained. "I have too much swelling and pain in my right hand."

What other factors should be considered?

What does the catheter need to do for the patient? See Figure 10-1 for a decision tool. To determine this, the nurse needs to first consider factors regarding the infusion (e.g., vesicant infusions, blood products, parenteral nutrition), high flow rates, and frequent CT scans, as well as pH level ($[< 5$ or $> 9]$, osmolarity > 600 mOsm/L, $> 10\%$ glucose). Other factors that should be considered include apheresis, dialysis, stem cell infusion, transfusion exchange, previous medical history, current laboratory results, and risk of infection related to catheter insertion and maintenance. Patient-specific

Figure 10-1. Vascular Access Choice Algorithm

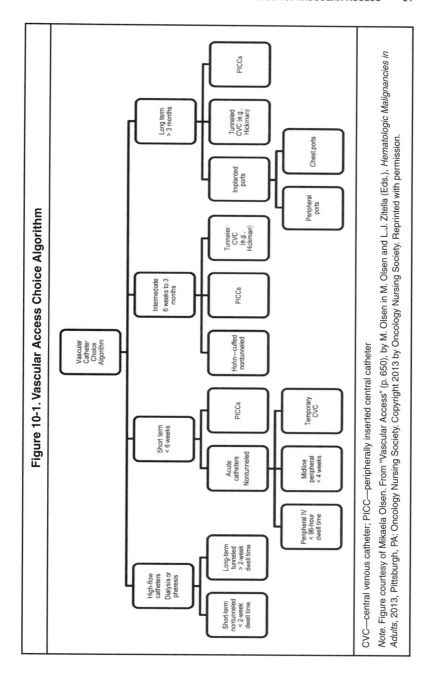

CVC—central venous catheter; PICC—peripherally inserted central catheter

Note. Figure courtesy of Mikaela Olsen. From "Vascular Access" (p. 650), by M. Olsen in M. Olsen and L.J. Zitella (Eds.), *Hematologic Malignancies in Adults*, 2013, Pittsburgh, PA: Oncology Nursing Society. Copyright 2013 by Oncology Nursing Society. Reprinted with permission.

considerations appear in Figure 10-2. Central line infection prevention strategies can be found in Figure 10-3.

Key Points
- Consider patient preference and past medical history.
- Place the smallest bore possible with the least number of lumens needed.
- Choose a central venous catheter if drug properties are contraindicated through a peripheral vein.
- Validate the patient's understanding of the catheter types.
- Choose a central venous catheter if a vesicant will be administered as a continuous infusion.

J.G. does not have a history of thrombus and is not on any medications except vitamin D. Laboratory values are as follows: platelet count = 280,000/mm^3, activated partial thromboplastin = 26.5 secs,

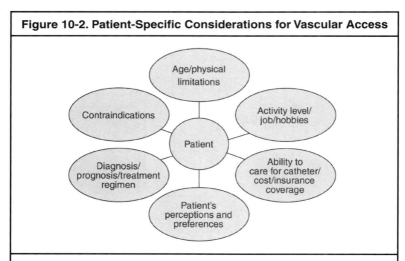

Figure 10-2. Patient-Specific Considerations for Vascular Access

Age/physical limitations

Contraindications

Activity level/ job/hobbies

Patient

Diagnosis/ prognosis/treatment regimen

Ability to care for catheter/ cost/insurance coverage

Patient's perceptions and preferences

Note. Based on information from Infusion Nurses Society, 2011.

From "Vascular Access" (p. 655), by M. Olsen in M. Olsen and L.J. Zitella (Eds.), *Hematologic Malignancies in Adults*, 2013, Pittsburgh, PA: Oncology Nursing Society. Copyright 2013 by Oncology Nursing Society. Reprinted with permission.

Figure 10-3. Central Line–Associated Bloodstream Infection Prevention Strategies

- Perform hand hygiene prior to any interaction with a central venous access device (CVAD).
- Use chlorhexidine for skin antisepsis.
- Avoid topical antimicrobial ointments (exception: dialysis catheters).
- Prevent colonization of hub of catheter: Scrub the hub before each access using strict aseptic technique.
- Cover catheter and catheter connections during showering.
- Change dressing routinely and whenever site is soiled, loose, or wet.
- Change tubing and needleless connectors using a strict schedule.
- Assess the need for CVAD daily and remove when no longer needed.

Note. Based on information from Furuya et al., 2011; Lopez, 2011; Murphy et al., 2010; O'Grady et al., 2011; Pronovost et al., 2006; Render et al., 2006.

---

prothrombin time = 10.4 secs, international normalized ratio = 0.9, and fibrinogen = 210 mg/dl.

Based on J.G.'s preferences and the information provided, what are his venous access options?

J.G. requires a CVAD because of the need for continuous-infusion vesicant chemotherapy. The catheter type options for J.G. include a peripherally inserted central catheter (PICC), an implanted chest wall tunneled central venous port, or a tunneled chest central venous catheter. J.G. has voiced concern about a catheter in his left arm and wishes to avoid a PICC at this time. He prefers to be free of any external lumens between treatments. J.G. verbalizes understanding of the need for needle sticks when accessing an implanted port prior to each treatment. He agrees to have an implanted port placed by interventional radiology providers before starting his chemotherapy treatment.

What education does J.G. need in order to care for his catheter?

Education for central catheter maintenance should include proper aseptic technique when performing dressing changes, cap changes, and flushing of the catheter. A focus on education related to catheter-related infection and thrombus, with strategies to minimize these risks, is crucial. J.G. should also be taught the importance of hygiene before handling the catheter. Activity limitations should also be reviewed with J.G.

Key Points

- Continuous infusions of vesicant chemotherapy must be infused through a central venous access device with a vigorous blood return because of the risk of extravasation and tissue damage.
- A central venous catheter tip should reside in the superior vena cava.
- Blood return should be verified per institutional policy when infusing continuous vesicant therapy.

J.G. receives his first two cycles of chemotherapy through his implanted port catheter without any problems. When attempting to obtain blood work, prior to his third cycle, the nurse notes that his catheter flushes well and does not have a blood return. The nurse instills 2 ml of 1:1,000 units/ml heparin, which dwells for 30 minutes. However, the catheter still does not exhibit a blood return. The catheter is easy to flush, the site is free of erythema and edema, and the patient denies any acute discomfort.

What can cause a catheter to lose a free-flowing brisk blood return upon aspiration?

This type of occlusion is most likely a partial occlusion. The assessment for occlusion starts at the bedside while troubleshooting the cause of little to no blood return. A visual assessment is performed to observe for swelling in the extremities. The nurse asks J.G. about any symptoms, such as new pain or numbness, or shortness of breath, syncope, chest pain, or heart palpitations since his last visit. A visual inspection of the catheter is necessary to rule out possible mechanical occlusions, such as kinks in the catheter tubing, issues with sutures, or damage to the catheter. As part of the catheter assessment, J.G. may change his position from sitting to standing or lying flat while flushing the catheter in an attempt to facilitate blood return. The patient may need to raise or cross his arms. He may need to turn his head away from the catheter and cough, breathe deeply, or perform a Valsalva maneuver to facilitate blood return. Any or all of these interventions are appropriate in the presence of flushing patency without discomfort. Tips for assessing and troubleshooting causes of mechanical occlusions can be found in Table 10-1. Although these previously mentioned nonpharmacologic strategies for troubleshooting occlusions are described and recommended in the literature, research is needed to determine their effectiveness (Mason, Ferrall, Boyington, & Reich, 2014).

Table 10-1. Management of Central Venous Catheter Mechanical Obstructions

Obstruction	Assessment Findings	Treatment
Crimping of tubing or catheter Clamp closed on patient side Clogged needleless connector Suture too tight Needleless securement device pinching catheter	Inability to flush or aspirate	Remove existing dressing to assess for kinks. Remove existing needleless connector and replace. Unclamp lumen.
Huber needle malposition	Absence of blood return Pain at implanted port site	Reposition or replace Huber needle and reassess for patency and blood return.
Implanted port rotation or flip	Malposition seen via chest x-ray (CXR) Possible broken or dislodged internal suture Inability to palpate port septum Pain and discomfort with access attempts	Consult interventional radiology to replace the internal sutures or replace the implanted port.
Catheter fracture	Edema and/or pain at catheter entry site or along tunnel Fluid leakage from the exit site	Obtain CXR. Perform cathetergram or dye flow study. Consult interventional radiology for removal.

(Continued on next page)

Table 10-1. Management of Central Venous Catheter Mechanical Obstructions *(Continued)*

Obstruction	Assessment Findings	Treatment
Catheter in right atrium	Chest pain Shortness of breath Heart palpitations	Obtain CXR. Reposition catheter tip back into superior vena cava.
Catheter tip in jugular	Earache on side of catheter Gurgling sound heard while catheter being flushed	Obtain CXR. Remove catheter or consult interventional radiology to reposition.
Embolization	Chest pain Shortness of breath Heart palpitations Neck or shoulder pain Edema	Consult interventional radiology for emergent catheter fragment removal.
Pinch-off syndrome (intermittent mechanical occlusion) Compression of catheter between first rib and clavicle Fractured catheter	May exhibit blood return with a position change (e.g., arm on catheter side above head) Possible signs of fracture or embolization.	Consult interventional radiology for removal. Assess catheter after removal to ensure it is intact.

Note. Based on information from Clark & Plaizier, 2011; Olsen, 2009.

What if the catheter cannot be flushed or aspirated?

This type of occlusion is called a complete withdrawal occlusion. Complete occlusions are difficult to manage and should be avoided by consistently ensuring patency of the catheter. An occluded catheter should never be flushed against resistance; this could result in catheter damage. Occlusions can be related to drug precipitate, intraluminal clotted blood, or fibrin formation, such as a fibrin sheath or fibrin tail. The occlusion of a CVAD is always considered an abnormal finding, and investigation into the underlying cause with prompt resolution of the problem should be initiated. Improper evaluation of an occluded catheter can lead to life-threatening catheter-related bloodstream infection, delay of treatment, and removal of the nonfunctioning catheter (Gaddh et al., 2014). Insertion of a new catheter can be costly and potentially risky for the patient. Figure 10-4 demonstrates a stopcock method for management of a complete withdrawal occlusion. This technique creates a vacuum in the catheter, allowing for the slow instillation of alteplase (Cummings-Winfield & Mushani-Kanji, 2008).

After mechanical or chemical occlusion is ruled out, a thrombus should be suspected. The treatment will consist of thrombolytic therapy or interventional radiology consultation. Accurate assessment and prompt intervention are crucial to properly identify the type of occlusion and initiate the interventions to correct the problem. The types of thrombotic occlusions are fibrin tail, fibrin sheath, mural thrombus, and intraluminal thrombus. These occlusions are pictured in Figure 10-5, along with nursing considerations, which are presented in Table 10-2.

Figure 10-4. Vacuum Technique for Instilling Alteplase With Complete Occlusion

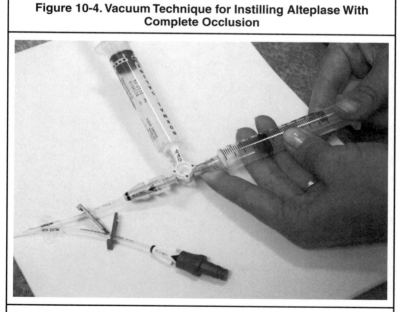

Note. Figure courtesy of Mikaela Olsen. Used with permission.

Figure 10-5. Types of Thrombotic Occlusions

| Fibrin tail | Fibrin sheath | Mural thrombus | Intraluminal thrombus |

Note. Figure courtesy of Genentech, Inc. Used with permission.

Table 10-2. Nursing Considerations for Thrombotic Occlusions

Description	Nursing Considerations
Intraluminal thrombi • Form inside the lumen of the catheter • 5%–25% of thrombotic occlusions • Partial or complete	If untreated, a partial thrombus may progress to a complete thrombus. Poor flushing technique after blood withdrawal promotes this type of thrombus. Perform declotting.
Mural thrombi • Caused by vessel trauma or previous vessel injury • Fibrin from the vessel-wall injury binds to cover the catheter surface.	Frequent cannulation attempts promote this type of thrombus. Rigid catheters increase the risk of a mural thrombus.
Fibrin sheath (see Figure 10-6) • Occurs in up to 47% of patients with central lines • Forms when fibrin adheres to the catheter's external surface forming a sock-like sheath • Can progress to cause catheter malfunction or a mural thrombus	Consider interventional radiology consult.
Fibrin tail • Forms when the catheter tip moves against the wall of the vein and fibrin attaches to the end of the catheter • The tail acts as a one-way valve, allowing fluid to infuse but preventing aspiration of blood. • Can progress to a total occlusion	If untreated, a partial thrombus may progress to a complete thrombus. Perform declotting.

Note. Based on information from Earhart, 2012.

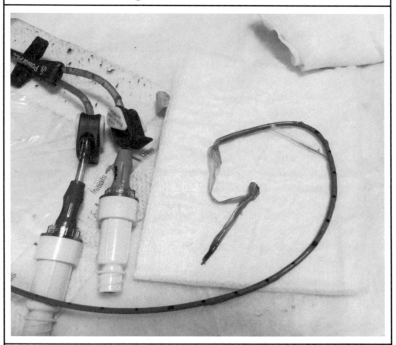

Figure 10-6. Fibrin Sheath

Note. Figure courtesy of Mikaela Olsen. Used with permission.

Key Points

- Heparin use prevents coagulation and deters fibrin formation; it should not be the treatment of choice for a catheter occlusion.
- Syringes that are 10 ml or larger are the safest size for flushing and withdrawing from a CVAD. Smaller syringes could cause potential rupture because of the increased pressure exerted (Infusion Nurses Society, 2011).
- The most common causes of absence of blood return are a result of mechanical, chemical, or thrombotic problems.

- Intraluminal occlusions can be partial or complete. Intraluminal occlusions result from inadequate flushing between medications or after drawing blood. Inadequate flushing can result in a buildup in the lumen, resulting in a sluggish or occluded catheter (Cummings-Winfield & Mushani-Kanji, 2008).
- Extraluminal occlusions (outside the lumen at the distal tip) can be partial or complete and usually involve fibrin accumulation, which affects both inward and outward flow (Cummings-Winfield & Mushani-Kanji, 2008).
- A chest x-ray (CXR) may be used to verify central line tip location, which may indicate a malposition or catheter defect and can result in the catheter malfunctioning.
- Once it has been determined that the occlusion is not mechanical, orders for the declotting protocol can be implemented.
- If the mechanical obstruction requires catheter repositioning or replacement, interventional radiology or a PICC RN should evaluate and treat as required.
- Prior to administration of chemotherapy, the central line should have a vigorous blood return.
- A CXR to verify tip location may be warranted if symptoms of catheter malposition are present.

After reviewing J.G.'s CXR (see Figure 10-7), it is determined that his implanted port is properly located in the superior vena cava. The nurse initiates the declotting protocol and instills alteplase per package insert. Alteplase dwells in J.G.'s port for 30 minutes, and the nurse is able to aspirate the alteplase and blood back into the syringe. She follows this with a 10 ml normal saline flush and is able to confirm patency of the catheter. J.G. receives the remaining cycles of chemotherapy without further occlusion problems.

Conclusion

The importance of evaluating and treating catheter occlusion should be underscored. Venous access assessment continues to be

Figure 10-7. Implanted Port X-Ray

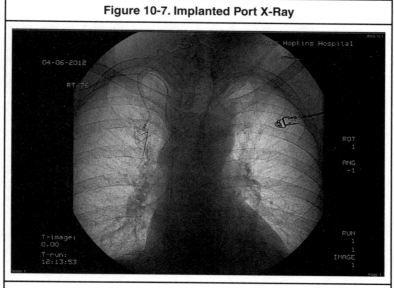

Note. Figure courtesy of MiKaela Olsen. Used with permission.

paramount in providing care for patients with devices. Improper catheter care and assessment can result in complete device occlusion, a major thrombotic event, superior vena catheter syndrome, infection, and, ultimately, the need to replace the access device. Ongoing catheter assessment with vigorous flushing after each use continues to be the key to occlusion prevention. In addition to these problems, J.G. was at risk for experiencing a treatment delay because of the occlusion.

References

Clark, D.K., & Plaizier, E. (2011). Devastating cerebral air embolism after central line removal. *Journal of Neuroscience Nursing, 43,* 193–196. doi:10.1097/JNN.0b013e3182212a3a

Cummings-Winfield, C., & Mushani-Kanji, T. (2008). Restoring patency to central venous access devices. *Clinical Journal of Oncology Nursing, 12,* 925–934. doi:10.1188/08.CJON.925-934

Earhart, A. (2012). Recognizing, preventing, and troubleshooting central-line complications. *American Nurse Today, 8*(11), 18–24. Retrieved from https://www

.americannursetoday.com/assets/0/434/436/440/10874/10876/10880/10942
/29ea8e71-23b2-45bc-90ac-43b0d6f19484.pdf

Elsevier Mosby. (2012). *Mosby's dictionary of medicine, nursing, and health professions* (9th ed.). St Louis, MO: Author.

Furuya, E.Y., Dick, A., Perencevich, E.N., Pogorzelska, M., Goldmann, D., & Stone, P.W. (2011). Central line bundle implementation in US intensive care units and impact on bloodstream infections. *PLOS ONE, 6*(1), e15452. doi:10.1371/journal.pone.0015452

Gaddh, M., Anton, A., Yamandia, K., Gupta, P., Tran, H., El Rassi, F., ... Khoury, H.J. (2014). Venous access catheter-related thrombosis in patients with cancer. *Leukemia and Lymphoma, 55*, 501–508. doi:10.3109/10428194.2013.813503

Infusion Nurses Society. (2011). Infusion nursing standards of practice. *Journal of Infusion Nursing, 34*, S1–S92.

Lopez, A.C. (2011). A quality improvement program combining maximum barrier precaution compliance monitoring and daily chlorhexidine gluconate baths resulting in decreased central line bloodstream infections. *Dimensions in Critical Care Nursing, 30*, 293–298. doi:10.1097/DCC.0b013e318227767f

Mason, T.M., Ferrall, S.M., Boyington, A.R., & Reich, R.R. (2014). Central venous access devices: An investigation of oncology nurses' troubleshooting techniques. *Clinical Journal of Oncology Nursing, 18*, 421–425. doi:10.1188/14.CJON.421-425

Murphy, D.J., Needham, D.M., Goeschel, C., Fan, E., Cosgrove, S.E., & Pronovost, P.J. (2010). Monitoring and reducing central line–associated bloodstream infections: A national survey of state hospital associations. *American Journal of Medical Quality, 25*, 255–260. doi:10.1177/1062860610364653

O'Grady, N., Alexander, M., Burns, L.A., Dellinger, E.P., Garland, J., Heard, S.O., ... Healthcare Infection Control Practices Advisory Committee. (2011). Guidelines for the prevention of intravascular catheter-related infections, 2011. Retrieved from http://www.cdc.gov/hicpac/pdf/guidelines/bsi-guidelines-2011.pdf

Olsen, M. (2009). Nursing-specific issues. In D. Ettinger, R. Donehower, R. Schwartz, & M. Olsen (Eds.), *Current cancer therapeutics* (5th ed., pp. 379–386). Philadelphia, PA: Springer.

Pronovost, P., Needham, D., Berenholtz, S., Sinopoli, D., Chu, H., Cosgrove, S., ... Goeschel, C. (2006). An intervention to decrease catheter-related bloodstream infections in the ICU. *New England Journal of Medicine, 355*, 2725–2732. doi:10.1056/NEJMoa061115

Render, M.L., Brungs, S., Kotagal, U., Nicholson, M., Burns, P., Ellis, D., ... Hirschhorn, L. (2006). Evidence-based practice to reduce central line infections. *Joint Commission Journal on Quality and Patient Safety, 32*, 253–260.

CASE 11
Patient Assessment and Dose Calculation

Michael Smart, RN, BSN, OCN®

A 65-year-old woman with lung cancer

C.K., a 65-year-old woman with a 40-pack-year smoking history, is referred to an oncologist for newly diagnosed metastatic non-small cell lung cancer. The cancer was discovered during hospitalization for pneumonia. Other comorbid conditions include diabetes with associated peripheral neuropathy and mild tinnitus.

During her initial meeting with the oncologist, C.K. mentions she is worried about the side effects of chemotherapy. Her father was treated for lung cancer in the 1980s, and she recalls nausea and vomiting being particularly problematic for him. She also says she heard that lung cancer can now be treated with a pill.

Can C.K.'s cancer be treated with an oral agent?

Erlotinib is an oral tyrosine kinase inhibitor that targets epidermal growth factor receptors (EGFRs) that are overexpressed in some lung cancers. For some tumors with specific EGFR mutations, erlotinib is an appropriate first-line treatment instead of standard chemotherapy (Khozin et al., 2014). Advantages include ease of dosing and convenience that the treatment comes in pill form. Patients who qualify start on 150 mg PO daily on an empty stomach. The most common adverse side effects include diarrhea and skin rash. The diarrhea is typically well managed with loperamide. Patients are advised to avoid sun exposure in order to limit severity of skin rashes (Astellas Pharma US, Inc., & Genentech, Inc., 2012). Unfortunately, based on the results of her EGFR mutation test, C.K. is not a candidate for erlotinib. Her physician recommends standard platinum-based doublet chemotherapy instead.

The decision is made to use cisplatin, a platinum agent, along with paclitaxel. Knowing that paclitaxel could worsen C.K.'s neuropathy, the oncologist orders carboplatin to minimize additional neurologic problems that might be caused by cisplatin. In addition to reduced renal toxicity, carboplatin also has lower emetogenic potential compared to cisplatin, which is very important to C.K. Carboplatin does cause prolonged cytopenias, and the oncology nurse will provide education that focuses on the problems associated with increased risk for infection and bleeding (Polovich, Olsen, & LeFebvre, 2014). The RN reassures C.K. that the goal is to prevent any chemotherapy-induced nausea and vomiting (CINV) and that additional measures will be taken immediately should nausea occur. Addressing C.K.'s anxieties related to CINV is, in itself, an important intervention to prevent CINV (Yap, Low, Chui, & Chan, 2012).

What is the treatment plan for C.K.?

C.K.'s treatment will consist of carboplatin AUC 5 and paclitaxel 200 mg/m^2 on day 1 of each three-week cycle for a total of four cycles. AUC, or "area under the curve," is a method of expressing drug exposure over time, and because the kidneys excrete carboplatin in a reliable manner, AUC is the optimal method to dose carboplatin in adults. Paclitaxel is dosed by using the more common approach of considering body surface area (BSA) (mg/m^2).

Complete chemotherapy orders include all the variables used to calculate the doses (e.g., height, weight, BSA, and renal function if applicable), as well as the final calculated patient-specific doses. Additionally, complete orders specify the route, rate, duration of infusion, date, and any necessary premedications (Neuss et al., 2013).

The oncology pharmacist verifies the physician's orders, and, according to the standard of care and institutional policy, the nurse performs an independent review and verification of the orders. This platinum doublet is commonly used by the physician, and the RN recognizes it as an appropriate regimen for treating lung cancer (National Comprehensive Cancer Network®, 2015).

To verify dosage calculations, the nurse needs to know the patient's age, gender, weight, height, and serum creatinine. The physician opts to estimate glomerular filtration rate (GFR) based on serum creatinine rather than perform a 24-hour urine collection. This is referred to as a calculated or estimated creatinine clearance (estCrCl).

The organization's policy for chemotherapy verification allows for a 10% variance between the planned dose and the actual dose to be administered before the RN must seek order clarification. This allows for small weight changes, differences in rounding, or difficulty in measuring small volumes and minimizes the need for new orders because of minor dose variations.

For example, if the planned dose for an accepted regimen is 50 mg/m² and the patient's BSA is 2 m², the planned dose is 100 mg (50 mg × 2 m²). The 10% variance rule allows 90–110 mg as an acceptable dose to be ordered. The utility of this can be seen with a planned dose calculation resulting in 99 mg. Rounding to 100 mg may make the dose more easily measured.

Because chemotherapy has a narrow therapeutic window and decisions regarding an appropriate variance are not in the scope of nursing practice, acceptable variance should be stated in policy (Polovich et al., 2014). Many organizations choose a more restrictive variance of 5%. Using the 100 mg example, 95–105 mg would be acceptable with a 5% variance rule.

RNs sometimes use a computer program that has been validated for accurately calculating information such as BSA, but they also need to know how to calculate these values using a calculator with a square root function.

What is C.K.'s planned dose for paclitaxel?

BSA is expressed in square meters (m²) and is usually calculated through the Mosteller equation by taking the square root of [height (cm) × weight (kg)/3,600] (Mosteller, 1987). If height and weight are measured in inches and pounds, BSA is still expressed in m² and is calculated by taking the square root of [height (in.) × weight (lbs)/3,131].

C.K. is 165 cm tall and weighs 70 kg. This is all that is needed to calculate the paclitaxel dose.

1. Using kilograms and centimeters to calculate BSA: the square root of [(165 cm × 70 kg)/3,600] = the square root of 3.2083 = 1.79 m²
2. 200 mg/m² × 1.79 m² = 358 mg is the planned dose.
3. The physician rounds the dosage to 350 mg, as allowed by policy.

4. With the 10% variance allowed by institutional policy, the RN confirms that the 350 mg dose is acceptable. The 10% variance rule allows a range of 322–394 mg. A 5% variance rule would allow 340–376 mg as acceptable doses.

Why use AUC instead of BSA for carboplatin dosing?

In preparing to verify the carboplatin dose, the nurse notes that C.K. is a 65-year-old woman who weighs 70 kg and has a serum creatinine of 0.4 mg/dl.

AUC is used to determine carboplatin doses instead of BSA. AUC is a method of expressing the intended exposure to the drug over time that accounts for renal function. However, different formulas can be used to determine renal function or GFR. Verification of carboplatin doses can be daunting if institutional policies are not clear regarding which formulas to use and under what conditions. In the absence of clear institutional direction, documentation in the orders and plan of care must state the process used to determine the intended dose.

The nurse notes that the Calvert formula was used to calculate C.K.'s carboplatin dose as per institutional policy. Using the Calvert formula (Polovich et al., 2014), the calculation is as follows:

$$\frac{\text{Carboplatin}}{\text{dose}} = \text{target AUC (mg/ml/min)} \times (\text{GFR} + 25)\,(\text{ml/min})$$

When a 24-hour urine is not used to measure GFR, the patient's age, gender, weight, and serum creatinine can be used to estimate CrCl instead, which is used in place of GFR. The RN notes that the physician wrote "estCrCl = 125." Using this value, the nurse calculates the intended carboplatin dose as follows:

$$5\ \text{mg/ml/min} \times (125 + 25)\ \text{ml/min} = 5 \times 150 = 750\ \text{mg}$$

This is the same dose the physician wrote in the chemotherapy orders. Initially, the nurse is confident the dose is correct, but a second nurse calculates the dose as 895 mg. The second nurse thinks the physician was wrong to use an estCrCl of 125 ml/min and should have used 155 ml/min instead. Is the second nurse right? No; however, the reason is not easily apparent without knowledge of recent changes in carboplatin dosing guidelines (Smart, 2011). The first nurse relied on the physician-documented estCrCl, which should have been independently verified.

Unless otherwise ordered, institutional policy requires using the Cockcroft-Gault method of estimating CrCl. With this formula, the calculation of estCrCl is as follows (Cockcroft & Gault, 1976):

Males:

$$\text{estCrCl (ml/min)} = \frac{(140 - age) \times (weight\ in\ kg)}{72 \times serum\ creatinine\ (mg/dl)}$$

Females:

$$\text{estCrCl (ml/min)} = \frac{(140 - age) \times (weight\ in\ kg) \times (0.85)}{72 \times serum\ creatinine\ (mg/dl)}$$

$$\text{estCrCl} = (140 - 65) \times 70 \times 0.85 / (72 \times 0.4)$$
$$\text{estCrCl} = (75 \times 70 \times 0.85) / (72 \times 0.4)$$
$$\text{estCrCl} = 4,462 / 29 = 154\ ml/min$$

So the second nurse calculated the carboplatin dose as follows:

$$5\ mg/ml/min \times (154 + 25)\ ml/min = 5 \times 179 = 895\ mg$$

What institutional policy did not account for (and neither RN was aware of) is the change in carboplatin dosing guidelines in 2010. This is a situation that illustrates the importance of keeping up to date on current standards of care. Although these calculations are useful to estimate CrCl, they are not without weakness. Formulas tend to overestimate CrCl in patients with a low (e.g., 0.4 mg/dl) serum creatinine and normal renal function. Using estCrCl without taking this into account can result in the patient receiving too much carboplatin. Because of toxicities without added benefit, the U.S. Food and Drug Administration issued guidelines stating that if estCrCl is used to calculate carboplatin doses, it should be capped at 125 ml/min (Smart, 2011).

Confusion could have also been avoided with clear documentation from the physician that a capped estCrCl was being used. Armed with this information obtained after discussion with the physician, the two nurses independently verify the correct dose of 750 mg for this patient, with estCrCl capped at 125 ml/min [5 × (125 + 50) = 5 × 150 = 750].

With all concerns addressed and premedications administered, the nurse checks off the chemotherapy at the patient's chairside with another qualified oncology nurse. C.K. tolerates her first cycle of chemotherapy without complications and is provided with discharge instructions; arrangements are made for her follow-up visit. Before her next appointment, C.K. expresses relief that her experience with chemotherapy is not what she had feared.

Key Points

- Have the patient's concerns (e.g., fear of nausea) been addressed?
- Is the regimen appropriate for disease being treated?
- Have independent dose calculations been verified?
- Are the variances within acceptable parameters?

Conclusion

Chemotherapy is an important tool in the fight against cancer, but chemotherapy also has a narrow therapeutic window. Give too little, and suboptimal therapeutic results can result. Give too much, and the patient is at risk for increased toxicity with no clinical benefit. The oncology nurse plays an important role in verifying the appropriateness of a prescribed regimen and the accuracy of dose calculations. The nurse is the last safety valve before the chemotherapy is given to the patient.

References

Astellas Pharma US, Inc., & Genentech, Inc. (2012). *Tarceva® (erlotinib)* [Package insert]. Retrieved from http://www.gene.com/download/pdf/tarceva_prescribing.pdf

Cockcroft, D.W., & Gault, M.H. (1976). Prediction of creatinine clearance from serum creatinine. *Nephron, 16*, 31–41. doi:10.1159/000180580

Khozin, S., Blumenthal, G.M., Jiang, X., He, K., Boyd, K., Murgo, A., ... Pazdur, R. (2014). U.S. Food and Drug Administration approval summary: Erlotinib for the first-line treatment of metastatic non-small cell lung cancer with epidermal growth factor receptor exon 19 deletions or exon 21 (L858R) substitution mutations. *Oncologist, 19*, 774–779. doi:10.1634/theoncologist.2014-0089

Mosteller, R.D. (1987). Simplified calculation of body-surface area. *New England Journal of Medicine, 317*, 1098. doi:10.1056/NEJM198710223171717

National Comprehensive Cancer Network. (2015). *NCCN Clinical Practice Guidelines in Oncology (NCCN Guidelines®): Non-small cell lung cancer* [v.4.2015]. Retrieved from http://www.nccn.org/professionals/physician_gls/pdf/nscl.pdf

Neuss, M.N., Polovich, M., McNiff, K., Esper, P., Gilmore, T., LeFebvre, K.B., ... Jacobson, J.O. (2013). 2013 updated American Society of Clinical Oncology/Oncology

Nursing Society chemotherapy administration safety standards including standards for the safe administration and management of oral chemotherapy. *Journal of Oncology Practice, 9*(25), 5s–13s. doi:10.1200/JOP.2013.000874

Polovich, M., Olsen, M., & LeFebvre, K.B. (Eds.). (2014). *Chemotherapy and biotherapy guidelines and recommendations for practice* (4th ed.). Pittsburgh, PA: Oncology Nursing Society.

Smart, M. (2011). Oncology update. *Oncology Nursing Forum, 38,* 93–94. doi:10.1188/11.ONF.93-94

Yap, K.Y., Low, X.H., Chui, W.K., & Chan, A. (2012). Computational prediction of state anxiety in Asian patients with cancer susceptible to chemotherapy-induced nausea and vomiting. *Journal of Clinical Psychopharmacology, 32,* 207–217. doi:10.1097/JCP.0b013e31824888a1

CASE 12
Infusion Reaction

Seth Eisenberg, RN, ASN, OCN®, BMTCN™

A 51-year-old woman with recurrent breast cancer

T.M., a 51-year-old woman with recurrent breast cancer, is scheduled to receive her first dose of paclitaxel. The nurse premedicates her with diphenhydramine, dexamethasone, and ranitidine in addition to antiemetics. The nurse reviews potential infusion-related side effects with T.M. and her husband, who has accompanied her to the appointment. After discussing side effects (e.g., chills, numbness, fever, increased blood pressure), the nurse starts the paclitaxel infusion.

Key Points

- Patients and family members should be familiar with signs and symptoms of hypersensitivity reaction (HSR) (Polovich, Olsen, & LeFebvre, 2014).
- Having medication and emergency equipment readily available to treat an HSR increases patient safety (Vogel, 2010).

Six minutes into the infusion, T.M. begins to experience mild itching on her neck and arms. She asks her husband to call for the nurse. When the nurse arrives, T.M. is tachypneic, with a respiratory rate of 28 breaths per min. She says she is itching and cannot seem to catch her breath. The nurse observes that she is having difficulty speaking. Her husband adds that she is also feeling dizzy and nauseated and having back pain.

What is the nurse's initial assessment?

T.M. is experiencing an HSR. *HSR* is a general term and includes those reactions classified as anaphylactic or anaphylactoid (also known as nonallergic), depending on the physiologic mechanisms involved (see Table 12-1). Historically, the Gell and Coombs model for allergic reactions defines anaphylaxis as being type I, immunoglobulin E (IgE)-mediated. These antibody-antigen reactions require prior exposure to the offending molecule (e.g., peanuts or cephalosporin) (Baldo & Pham, 2013; Ben-Shoshan & Clarke, 2011; Descotes & Choquet-Kastylevsky, 2001). However, HSR occurring with the first dose of a medication, as in T.M.'s case, is typically not the result of the presence of antibodies. Regardless of the etiology, the signs and symptoms of anaphylactoid HSRs are often indis-

Table 12-1. Anaphylactoid/CARPA Versus Anaphylactic Reactions

Characteristic	Anaphylactoid/CARPA	Anaphylaxis (Antibody Dependent)
Initiating mechanism	Non-IgG- or IgE-dependent, with subsequent complement activation and mast cell degranulation	IgG- or IgE-dependent, with subsequent mast cell degranulation with or without complement activation
Prior exposure	Not required	Required (except with cross-reactivity)
Subsequent therapy	HSRs decrease with subsequent doses.	HSRs worsen with subsequent doses.
Frequency	Relatively common in oncology	Relatively rare in oncology
Resolution	HSRs can resolve with or without treatment but may progress to requiring treatment.	HSRs will always require treatment.
Rechallenge	Can be rechallenged if HSR is mild. Desensitization may be an option.	Even mild HSRs should not be rechallenged, although desensitization may be an option.

CARPA—complement activation–related pseudoallergy; HSR—hypersensitivity reaction; IgE—immunoglobulin E; IgG—immunoglobulin G

Note. Based on information from Baldo & Pham, 2013; Brown et al., 2013; Cernadas et al., 2010; Guitart, 2014; Mezzano et al., 2014; Stone et al., 2014; Szebeni, 2005.

to secondary agents, which are less effective and take longer to work (Simons et al., 2011).
- The normal adult dose of epinephrine is 0.3 mg of 1:1,000 concentration.
- The general consensus among allergy experts is that during an anaphylactic/anaphylactoid event, no contraindications to epinephrine are evident, and the life-saving benefits outweigh any potential risks (Sampson et al., 2005).
- The IM route is preferred over the subcutaneous (SC) route because of superior onset of action from epinephrine's ability to promote venous dilation in skeletal muscle (Lieberman et al., 2010; Simons, 2010).
- Epinephrine promotes bronchial relaxation by decreasing bronchospasm and dyspnea. Other beneficial effects include decreasing angioedema, gastrointestinal symptoms, and epidermal symptoms (e.g., itching, redness, wheals) (Mylan Specialty LP, 2012).
- Ensure the needle used for the administration of epinephrine is of sufficient length to penetrate the SC tissues (Lieberman et al., 2010).
- The use of prefilled epinephrine autoinjectors (e.g., EpiPen® Auto-Injector) saves valuable time and prevents medication errors that might occur in a crisis situation (Simons, 2010).
- Staff expected to use autoinjectors must be properly trained in order to avoid inadvertent needlestick injuries.
- After epinephrine administration, the patient should remain supine to prevent circulatory collapse associated with empty ventricle syndrome (Simons, 2010).

After three minutes, T.M.'s respiratory rate slows to 24 breaths per min, and she states that she is breathing easier. Her blood pressure is now 112/66 mm Hg, which is close to her preinfusion baseline. Oxygen saturation is now 98%, the wheezing has stopped, and the supplemental oxygen is discontinued. T.M.'s physician decides to admit her to the hospital for observation.

Key Points

- Careful monitoring is required after treatment of an HSR, and additional doses of epinephrine may be warranted if symptoms recur (Polovich et al., 2014).
- Patients may complain of headache and develop a mild tremor after epinephrine administration. The nurse should explain to the patient and family that these are common, expected short-term side effects.

T.M. is transported from the ambulatory clinic to the hospital with stable vital signs. T.M.'s physician informs her that, because of the severity of her reaction, he will select another therapy to treat her disease.

Conclusion

In T.M.'s case, the administration of paclitaxel resulted in a severe HSR. Signs and symptoms included profound hypotension, oxygen desaturation with respiratory distress, pruritus, and nausea. Prompt identification and management of an HSR is crucial. T.M.'s nurse discontinued the infusion and placed her in the Trendelenburg position. Upon arrival of the physician, she administered a normal saline bolus and a single dose of IM epinephrine. T.M.'s symptoms quickly resolved, and she was safely transported to the hospital.

References

Abraham, S.N., & St. John, A.L. (2010). Mast cell-orchestrated immunity to pathogens. *Nature Reviews Immunology, 10,* 440–452. doi:10.1038/nri2782

Baldo, B.A., & Pham, N.H. (2013). Adverse reactions to targeted and non-targeted chemotherapeutic drugs with emphasis on hypersensitivity responses and the invasive metastatic switch. *Cancer and Metastasis Reviews, 32,* 723–761. doi:10.1007/s10555-013-9447-3

Ben-Shoshan, M., & Clarke, A.E. (2011). Anaphylaxis: Past, present and future. *Allergy, 66,* 1–14. doi:10.1111/j.1398-9995.2010.02422.x

Boulanger, J., Boursiquot, J.N., Cournoyer, G., Lemieux, J., Masse, M.S., Almanric, K., ... Comité de l'évolution des pratiques en oncologie. (2014). Management of hypersensitivity to platinum- and taxane-based chemotherapy: CEPO review and clinical recommendations. *Current Oncology, 21,* e630–eE641. doi:10.3747/co.21.1966

Brown, S.G., Stone, S.F., Fatovich, D.M., Burrows, S.A., Holdgate, A., Celenza, A., … Isbister, G.K. (2013). Anaphylaxis: Clinical patterns, mediator release, and severity. *Journal of Allergy and Clinical Immunology, 132,* 1141–1149. doi:10.1016/j.jaci.2013.06.015

Carroll, M.V., & Sim, R.B. (2011). Complement in health and disease. *Advanced Drug Delivery Reviews, 63,* 965–975. doi:10.1016/j.addr.2011.06.005

Cernadas, J.R., Brockow, K., Romano, A., Aberer, W., Torres, M.J., Bircher, A., … European Network of Drug Allergy and the EAACI interest group on drug hypersensitivity. (2010). General considerations on rapid desensitization for drug hypersensitivity—A consensus statement. *Allergy, 65,* 1357–1366. doi:10.1111/j.1398-9995.2010.02441.x

Commins, S.P., Borish, L., & Steinke, J.W. (2010). Immunologic messenger molecules: Cytokines, interferons, and chemokines. *Journal of Allergy and Clinical Immunology, 125*(Suppl. 2), S53–S72. doi:10.1016/j.jaci.2009.07.008

Descotes, J., & Choquet-Kastylevsky, G. (2001). Gell and Coombs's classification: Is it still valid? *Toxicology, 158,* 43–49. doi:10.1016/S0300-483X(00)00400-5

Dye, D., & Watkins, J. (1980). Suspected anaphylactic reaction to Cremophor EL. *BMJ, 280,* 1353. doi:10.1136/bmj.280.6228.1353

Falcone, F.H., Haas, H., & Gibbs, B.F. (2000). The human basophil: A new appreciation of its role in immune responses. *Blood, 96,* 4028–4038.

Gelderblom, H., Verweij, J., Nooter, K., & Sparreboom, A. (2001). Cremophor EL: The drawbacks and advantages of vehicle selection for drug formulation. *European Journal of Cancer, 37,* 1590–1598. doi:10.1016/S0959-8049(01)00171-X

Guitart, M.C.C. (2014). Rapid drug desensitization for hypersensitivity reactions to chemotherapy and monoclonal antibodies in the 21st century. *Journal of Investigational Allergology and Clinical Immunology, 24,* 72–79. Retrieved from http://www.jiaci.org/issues/vol24issue2/vol24issue02-1.htm

Haroon, E., Raison, C.L., & Miller, A.H. (2012). Psychoneuroimmunology meets neuropsychopharmacology: Translational implications of the impact of inflammation on behavior. *Neuropsychopharmacology, 37,* 137–162. doi:10.1038/npp.2011.205

Hogan, A.D., & Schwartz, L.B. (1997). Markers of mast cell degranulation. *Methods, 13,* 43–52. doi:10.1006/meth.1997.0494

Kloover, J.S., den Bakker, M.A., Gelderblom, H., & van Meerbeeck, J.P. (2004). Fatal outcome of a hypersensitivity reaction to paclitaxel: A critical review of premedication regimens. *British Journal of Cancer, 90,* 304–305. doi:10.1038/sj.bjc.6601303

Lieberman, P., Nicklas, R.A., Oppenheimer, J., Kemp, S.F., Lang, D.M., Bernstein, D.I., … Wallace, D. (2010). The diagnosis and management of anaphylaxis practice parameter: 2010 update. *Journal of Allergy and Clinical Immunology, 126,* 477–480. doi:10.1016/j.jaci.2010.06.022

Markman, M., Kennedy, A., Webster, K., Kulp, B., Peterson, G., & Belinson, J. (2000). Paclitaxel-associated hypersensitivity reactions: Experience of the gynecologic oncology program of the Cleveland Clinic Cancer Center. *Journal of Clinical Oncology, 18,* 102–105.

Mezzano, V., Giavina-Bianchi, P., Picard, M., Caiado, J., & Castells, M. (2014). Drug desensitization in the management of hypersensitivity reactions to monoclonal antibodies and chemotherapy. *BioDrugs: Clinical Immunotherapeutics, Biopharmaceuticals and Gene Therapy, 28*, 133–144. doi:10.1007/s40259-013-0066-x

Moghimi, S.M., Andersen, A.J., Ahmadvand, D., Wibroe, P.P., Andresen, T.L., & Hunter, A.C. (2011). Material properties in complement activation. *Advanced Drug Delivery Reviews, 63*, 1000–1007. doi:10.1016/j.addr.2011.06.002

Mylan Specialty LP. (2012). *EpiPen®︎ (epinephrine)* [Package insert]. Basking Ridge, NJ: Author.

Netea, M.G., Kullberg, B.J., & Van der Meer, J.W. (2000). Circulating cytokines as mediators of fever. *Clinical Infectious Diseases, 31*(Suppl. 5), S178–S184. doi:10.1086/317513

Ono, E., Taniguchi, M., Mita, H., Fukutomi, Y., Higashi, N., Miyazaki, E., ... Akiyama, K. (2009). Increased production of cysteinyl leukotrienes and prostaglandin D2 during human anaphylaxis. *Clinical and Experimental Allergy, 39*, 72–80. doi:10.1111/j.1365-2222.2008.03104.x

Ortonne, J.P. (2012). Urticaria and its subtypes: The role of second-generation antihistamines. *European Journal of Internal Medicine, 23*, 26–30. doi:10.1016/j.ejim.2011.09.008

Pichler, W.J., Adam, J., Daubner, B., Gentinetta, T., Keller, M., & Yerly, D. (2010). Drug hypersensitivity reactions: Pathomechanism and clinical symptoms. *Medical Clinics of North America, 94*, 645–664, xv. doi:10.1016/j.mcna.2010.04.003

Polovich, M., Olsen, M., & LeFebvre, K.B. (Eds.). (2014). *Chemotherapy and biotherapy guidelines and recommendations for practice* (4th ed.). Pittsburgh, PA: Oncology Nursing Society.

Samlowski, W.E., Kondapaneni, M., Tharkar, S., McGregor, J.R., Laubach, V.E., & Salvemini, D. (2011). Endothelial nitric oxide synthase is a key mediator of interleukin-2-induced hypotension and vascular leak syndrome. *Journal of Immunotherapy, 34*, 419–427. doi:10.1097/CJI.0b013e31821dcb50

Sampson, H.A., Muñoz-Furlong, A., Bock, S.A., Schmitt, C., Bass, R., Chowdhury, B.A., ... Camargo, C.A., Jr. (2005). Symposium on the definition and management of anaphylaxis: Summary report. *Journal of Allergy and Clinical Immunology, 115*, 584–591. doi:10.1016/j.jaci.2005.01.009

Schwartz, J.R. (2012). Dexamethasone premedication for prophylaxis of taxane toxicities: Can the doses be reduced when paclitaxel or docetaxel are given weekly? *Journal of Oncology Pharmacy Practice, 18*, 250–256. doi:10.1177/1078155211409473

Simons, F.E. (2010). Anaphylaxis. *Journal of Allergy and Clinical Immunology, 125*(Suppl. 2), 161–181. doi:10.1016/j.jaci.2009.12.981

Simons, F.E.R., Ardusso, L.R.F., Bilò, M.B., El-Gamal, Y.M., Ledford, D.K., Ring, J., ... Thong, B.Y. (2011). World Allergy Organization anaphylaxis guidelines: Summary. *Journal of Allergy and Clinical Immunology, 127*, 587–593. doi:10.1016/j.jaci.2011.01.038

Singla, A.K., Garg, A., & Aggarwal, D. (2002). Paclitaxel and its formulations. *International Journal of Pharmaceutics, 235*, 179–192. doi:10.1016/S0378-5173(01)00986-3

Stone, S.F., Phillips, E.J., Wiese, M.D., Heddle, R.J., & Brown, S.G. (2014). Immediate-type hypersensitivity drug reactions. *British Journal of Clinical Pharmacology, 78*, 1–13. doi:10.1111/bcp.12297

Szebeni, J. (2005). Complement activation-related pseudoallergy: A new class of drug-induced acute immune toxicity. *Toxicology, 216*, 106–121. doi:10.1016/j.tox.2005.07.023

Vogel, W.H. (2010). Infusion reactions: Diagnosis, assessment, and management [Online exclusive]. *Clinical Journal of Oncology Nursing, 14,* E10–E21. doi:10.1188/10.CJON.E10-E21

Wang, H., Wang, H.S., & Liu, Z.P. (2011). Agents that induce pseudo-allergic reaction. *Drug Discoveries and Therapeutics, 5,* 211–219. doi:10.5582/ddt.2011.v5.5.211

Weiss, R.B., Donehower, R.C., Wiernik, P.H., Ohnuma, T., Gralla, R.J., Trump, D.L., ... Leyland-Jones, B. (1990). Hypersensitivity reactions from Taxol. *Journal of Clinical Oncology, 8,* 1263–1268.

Weiszhár, Z., Czúcz, J., Révész, C., Rosivall, L., Szebeni, J., & Rozsnyay, Z. (2012). Complement activation by polyethoxylated pharmaceutical surfactants: Cremophor-EL, Tween-80 and Tween-20. *European Journal of Pharmaceutical Sciences, 45,* 492–498. doi:10.1016/j.ejps.2011.09.016

Welle, M. (1997). Development, significance, and heterogeneity of mast cells with particular regard to the mast cell-specific proteases chymase and tryptase. *Journal of Leukocyte Biology, 61,* 233–245.

Zetka, E.S. (2012). The essentials of chemotherapy-induced infusion reactions. *Clinical Journal of Oncology Nursing, 16,* 527–529. doi:10.1188/12.CJON.527-529

CASE 13
Desensitization

Joshua Carter, BSN, RN, and Marlon Garzo Saria, MSN, RN, AOCNS®, FAAN

A 50-year-old woman requiring desensitization to carboplatin

M.P. is a 50-year-old woman with recurrent stage IIIC ovarian cancer who presents to the infusion center for her third cycle of single-agent carboplatin. This cycle follows a six-month platinum-free interval and three previous carboplatin treatment courses. After her initial tumor debulking nine years ago, M.P. completed six cycles of carboplatin and paclitaxel; three years later, she completed six cycles of gemcitabine and carboplatin and then 12 cycles of single-agent carboplatin, which was three years after her last carboplatin-containing regimen. She resumed a 12-cycle carboplatin course following a 10-month chemotherapy holiday.

What therapeutic options are available for relapsed ovarian carcinoma?

A combination of a platinum and taxane is considered the standard first-line therapy option for advanced-stage ovarian carcinoma as well as in the relapse setting. Carboplatin is equally as effective as cisplatin and has a more favorable toxicity profile; however, it carries a higher risk of a severe hypersensitivity reaction (HSR) (Pandey et al., 2014).

How common is carboplatin-induced hypersensitivity reaction?

Increased use of platinum agents has been associated with an increased occurrence of HSRs. For this particular class of antineoplastic agents, hypersensitivity is rarely reported during the initial course of treatment, but reactions can occur after multiple infusions with

113

no prior clinical signs. Carboplatin-based regimens are often administered over six cycles, and HSRs are more likely observed during retreatment following a period of remission (Boulanger et al., 2014). The reported incidence of HSR to carboplatin is 27% in patients who received more than seven treatments compared to 1% in patients who received fewer than six treatments (Banerji et al., 2014).

Key Points

- The majority (75%) of patients with recent history of HSR to carboplatin are more likely to have a severe reaction if rechallenged without desensitization (Pandey et al., 2014).
- Carboplatin desensitization is used in place of single-agent cisplatin, as it is better tolerated, with lower incidence of neurotoxicity, nephrotoxicity, and acute and delayed emesis (Pagani, 2010).

M.P. completed her 24th cycle of single-agent carboplatin without experiencing an HSR. She was responding well to the regimen, as evidenced by a stable computed tomography (CT) scan with no evidence of progression and normal cancer antigen (CA) 125. Three months later, however, her CA-125 and CT scan demonstrated disease progression. At that time, the oncologist recommended that she resume chemotherapy with her 25th carboplatin cycle while using a desensitization protocol.

What is desensitization?

Desensitization is a procedure used to reduce the severity and occurrence of allergic reactions during the course of chemotherapy. It involves "inducing a temporary tolerance to a treatment by gradually reintroducing a small amount of the antigen over a relatively short period of time until the total scheduled dose has been administered" (Boulanger et al., 2014, p. e634).

Who benefits from desensitization?

Desensitization is indicated when no alternative therapy is available or when the alternative therapy is less effective or more toxic than the treatment being used (Boulanger et al., 2014). It is also indicated in patients with a history of severe HSRs despite premedication or for select individuals who have had positive results in skin tests (Pagani, 2010).

Key Points

- Desensitization protocols should only be carried out by trained medical personnel with experience managing HSRs in a setting where emergency medication and monitoring equipment are available.
- Desensitization protocols can be used in the case of positive skin allergy tests to platinum drugs or prior severe HSR if substitution of treatment would affect patient survival (Boulanger et al., 2014).
- Desensitization protocols do not alter the effect of therapy (Pagani, 2010).

How is desensitization carried out in practice?

The most widely used desensitization protocol is the 12-step protocol, developed by the Dana-Farber Cancer Institute and Brigham and Women's Hospital. The protocol involves the preparation of three different dilutions of the drug, titrated using a 100-fold dilution (bag #1) of the final target concentration, a 10-fold dilution (bag #2), and the usual concentration of the drug (bag #3). The infusion rate is increased every 15 minutes, with the volume infused approximately double from the preceding step (Boulanger et al., 2014; Castells et al., 2008). Recently, a retrospective study by Takase et al. (2015) reported that more than 80% of patients using a four-step four-hour carboplatin desensitization protocol were able to complete the planned cycles. Of those who completed the planned cycles, 80% achieved disease control. In a patient with platinum-sensitive relapse, as in M.P.'s case, the treatment team might consider desensitization of carboplatin, as it can reduce subsequent HSRs (Pandey et al., 2014).

M.P. was premedicated with dexamethasone 20 mg IV, diphenhydramine 50 mg IV, and famotidine 20 mg IV 30 minutes prior to the start of the infusion. She tolerated the first bag (9 mg) of the desensitization well. However, she began experiencing flushing in the face, ears, and under the chin when the rate was increased during the second bag to the maximum rate of 40 ml/hr. She denied tingling in the lips or tongue, fullness in the throat, shortness of breath, chest pain or pressure, back pain, pruritus, or rash. She admitted to very mild abdominal tightness in a band-like distribution across the middle abdomen without nausea or cramping.

M.P. had a mild infusion reaction during carboplatin desensitization at the very end of bag #2. The infusion was immediately stopped, and normal saline was initiated. The advanced practice nurse ordered diphenhydramine 25 mg IV and then discussed the case with the oncologist. The oncologist requested hydrocortisone 50 mg IV and a one-hour monitoring period before rechallenging at half the rate (20 ml/hr for 15 minutes before 40 ml/hr for 15 minutes). The patient tolerated the rechallenge and completed bag #2 without further event. Bag #3 was titrated per the usual orders, and she made it through the 80 ml/hr maximum rate for 15 minutes before noting palmar pruritus. The infusion was stopped, and she was given another dose of diphenhydramine 25 mg IV and famotidine 20 mg IV. She then noted fullness in bilateral ears and nose as well as bilateral palmar edema. She was given a repeat dose of hydrocortisone 50 mg IV but still developed full-body urticaria. The case was discussed with the oncologist, who decided to discontinue the remaining dose of carboplatin. M.P. was monitored for an additional 90 minutes after complete resolution of symptoms.

Key Points

- The patient's safety is of utmost importance, and depending on the severity of the reaction, the provider may decide to discontinue treatment.
- Institutional policy differs widely, and medical personnel should be familiar with all orders of desensitization prior to administering chemotherapy.
- Patients should be educated to recognize the initial symptoms of hypersensitivity and to immediately inform medical personnel (Boulanger et al., 2014).

How are reactions managed during desensitization?

As with any other acute infusion-related reaction, immediately stop the infusion and maintain IV access using normal saline solution. Administer diphenhydramine or hydroxyzine 25–50 mg IV; famotidine 20 mg IV or ranitidine 50 mg IV; and methylprednisolone sodium succinate 0.5 mg/kg IV. Consider administering oxygen and nebulized albuterol if the patient exhibits respiratory symptoms. Epinephrine 0.3 ml (1 mg/ml) must be available at the bedside prior to the start of desensitization. Once the patient is stable and symptoms have resolved, resume the protocol, with physician approval, from the step at which it had been stopped (Castells et al., 2008).

Castells et al. (2008) reported that 7% of reactions occurred during the infusion of bag #1, 18% during infusion of bag #2, and 75% during infusion of bag #3. A majority of the reactions in patients who have received multiple desensitizations occurred during the first two procedures, with the frequency and severity of reactions declining with subsequent courses.

Key Points

- Emergency medications, including epinephrine, H_1 and H_2 antihistamines, bronchodilators, and oxygen, should be readily available during desensitization (Boulanger et al., 2014).
- Infusion should be immediately stopped when any signs or symptoms of infusion-related reaction are observed, and normal saline should be initiated. The provider will decide which medications will be given depending on the severity of symptoms.
- Retreatment with carboplatin for relapse of neoplasm is the strongest predictor of HSRs (Pagani, 2010).

Because M.P.'s recent imaging and CA-125 were suggestive of progression, her oncologist recommended that she continue with a platinum-based chemotherapy regimen. Unfortunately, she has had two reactions with the last two cycles of carboplatin using a desensitization protocol, with her last HSR being more severe than the first. M.P. agreed with her oncologist that she cannot continue with carboplatin. She was restarted with single-agent cisplatin because her disease has been very responsive to a platinum-based chemotherapy.

Conclusion

Carboplatin was recommended for M.P.'s case of recurrent stage IIIC, platinum-sensitive ovarian cancer. She had a long history of prior carboplatin exposure, and her physician thought it was best to use a desensitization protocol to prevent HSR. Unfortunately, M.P. was unable to tolerate the desensitization and was switched to a new therapy.

References

Banerji, A., Lax, T., Guyer, A., Hurwitz, S., Camargo, C.A., Jr., & Long, A.A. (2014). Management of hypersensitivity reactions to carboplatin and paclitaxel in an outpatient oncology infusion center: A 5-year review. *Journal of Allergy and Clinical Immunology, 2,* 428–433. doi:10.1016/j.jaip.2014.04.010

Boulanger, J., Boursiquot, J.N., Cournoyer, G., Lemieux, J., Masse, M.S., Almanric, K., ... Comité de l'évolution des pratiques en oncologie. (2014). Management of hypersensitivity to platinum- and taxane-based chemotherapy: CEPO review and clinical recommendations. *Current Oncology, 21,* e630–e641. doi:10.3747/co.21.1966

Castells, M.C., Tennant, N.M., Sloane, D.E., Hsu, F.I., Barrett, N.A., Hong, D.I., ... Matulonis, U.A. (2008). Hypersensitivity reactions to chemotherapy: Outcomes and safety of rapid desensitization in 413 cases. *Journal of Allergy and Clinical Immunology, 122,* 574–580. doi:10.1016/j.jaci.2008.02.044

Pagani, M. (2010). The complex clinical picture of presumably allergic side effects to cytostatic drugs: Symptoms, pathomechanism, reexposure, and desensitization. *Medical Clinics of North America, 94,* 835–852, xiii. doi:10.1016/j.mcna.2010.03.002

Pandey, A., Bhosale, B., Pandita, V., Singh, A., Ghosh, J., Ghosh, J., & Bajpai, J. (2014). Carboplatin hypersensitivity in relapsed ovarian carcinoma: A therapeutic challenge. *Indian Journal of Medical and Paediatric Oncology, 35,* 17–20. doi:10.4103/0971-5851.133705

Takase, N., Matsumoto, K., Onoe, T., Kitao, A., Tanioka, M., Kikukawa, Y., ... Negoro, S. (2015). 4-step 4-h carboplatin desensitization protocol for patients with gynecological malignancies showing platinum hypersensitivity: A retrospective study. *International Journal of Clinical Oncology, 20,* 566–573. doi:10.1007/s10147-014-0731-1

CASE 14
Extravasation

Daniel A. MacManus, RN, MSN, MBA, OCN®, CCRC

A 28-year-old woman with vesicant extravasation

L.B. is a 28-year-old woman with stage IVB Hodgkin lymphoma who presents to the infusion center for cycle 2, day 15 of doxorubicin, bleomycin, vinblastine, and dacarbazine (ABVD). She had already received the bleomycin and doxorubicin when she complains of a "cramping" sensation around her implanted port on her right upper anterior chest. Vinblastine is being administered via a steady IV drip as a secondary infusion and is about halfway into the 10-minute administration when the patient reports discomfort. She relates having some type of discomfort during her three previous treatments but states that this incident is the most intense. L.B. also has back pain and took oxycodone, which was previously prescribed for this underlying condition.

What can cause discomfort around the port site during infusion of ABVD?

The nurse considers the timing and location of discomfort during the infusion of ABVD and immediately suspects extravasation. Extravasation is the leakage of a vesicant into tissue or extravascular space around the infusion site (Al-Benna, O'Boyle, & Holley, 2013; Boschi & Rostagno, 2012; Clark et al., 2013; Pérez Fidalgo et al., 2012). This may occur as direct leakage from the venous access device or from elsewhere in the vessel (e.g., previous venipuncture).

Signs and symptoms of extravasation include tingling, burning, pain, swelling, pruritus, and redness at the injection site, which may manifest later (see Table 14-1) (Al-Benna et al., 2013; Pérez

Table 14-1. Signs and Symptoms of Vesicant Extravasation, Venous Irritation, and Flare Reaction

Signs and Symptoms	Vesicant Extravasation	Venous Irritation	Flare Reaction
Pain	Immediate: Pain typically occurs and is described as burning, stinging, or coolness at and around the vesicant administration site. However, pain may not always be present. Delayed: Pain usually increases in intensity over time.	Aching and tightness along a peripheral vein, above the administration site, occurs as the drug infuses.	No pain is present; the skin overlying the vein may itch.
Redness	Immediate: Redness in area of administration is common but is not always present or may be difficult to detect if extravasation occurs deeper in the tissue (e.g., resulting from needle displacement or dislodgment from implanted port). Delayed: Redness typically intensifies over time.	The vein may appear reddened or darkened.	Immediate blotches or streaks develop along the vein that usually subside within a few minutes. Wheals may appear along the vein.
Swelling	Immediate: Swelling is easier to see and detect when extravasation is superficial (e.g., from peripheral vein) rather than deeper in the tissue (e.g., implanted port). Delayed: Swelling generally increases over time.	Swelling does not occur.	Swelling does not occur.

(Continued on next page)

Table 14-1. Signs and Symptoms of Vesicant Extravasation, Venous Irritation, and Flare Reaction *(Continued)*

Signs and Symptoms	Vesicant Extravasation	Venous Irritation	Flare Reaction
Blood return	Immediate: Loss of blood return from IV device occurs.	Blood return should be present. If loss of blood return occurs, suspect infiltration of irritant.	Blood return is present.
Ulceration	Immediate: Skin integrity is intact. Delayed: If extravasation is not treated, blistering and sloughing begin within 1–2 weeks, followed by tissue necrosis that may require surgical debridement and skin grafting or flap placement.	Ulceration does not occur.	Ulceration does not occur.

Note. Based on information from Al-Benna et al., 2013; Goolsby & Lombardo, 2006; Pérez Fidalgo et al., 2012; Pikó et al., 2013; Sauerland et al., 2006; Schulmeister, 2011.

From *Chemotherapy and Biotherapy Guidelines and Recommendations for Practice* (4th ed., p. 157), by M. Polovich, M. Olsen, and K.B. LeFebvre (Eds.), 2014, Pittsburgh, PA: Oncology Nursing Society. Copyright 2014 by Oncology Nursing Society. Adapted with permission.

Fidalgo et al., 2012; Pikó et al., 2013). Additional late signs and symptoms can include blistering, mottling or darkening of the skin, firm induration, necrosis, and desquamation (Al-Benna et al., 2013). Indices of suspicion for extravasation include absence of blood return, resistance on the syringe plunger during delivery of an IV push drug, or interruption in the free flow of an infusion (Pérez Fidalgo et al., 2012). If extravasation is suspected, immediate action by the nurse can help prevent further complications (see Figure 14-1). L.B.'s nurse notes brisk blood return upon aspiration every two minutes during the infusion but stops the infusion anyway.

Figure 14-1. Steps in Managing a Suspected Extravasation

1. Immediately stop administering the vesicant and IV fluids.
2. Disconnect the IV tubing from the IV device. Do not remove the IV device or noncoring port needle.
3. Attempt to aspirate residual vesicant from the IV device or port needle using a small (1–3 ml) syringe. Remove the peripheral IV device or port needle.
4. Assess the site of the suspected extravasation.
5. Assess signs and symptoms experienced by the patient (e.g., pain, impairment in range of motion of extremity).
6. Notify the physician, physician assistant, or advanced practice nurse.
7. Initiate appropriate management measures in accordance with institutional policies.

Key Points

- Patients should be educated about risks of extravasation.
- Staff administering chemotherapy must receive adequate training in extravasation recognition and management.
- Nurses should monitor patients and vascular access sites for signs and symptoms of extravasation.
- Patients should be asked to immediately report any sensation of pain, tightening, burning, or any other unusual local sensation.
- Pain medications may mask the signs and symptoms of extravasation.

Physical assessment demonstrates a well-appearing woman in no acute distress resting comfortably in her chair. A port is located in the right upper anterior chest wall without signs of erythema, induration, venous discoloration, ecchymosis, subcutaneous edema, warmth, or discharge. The patient reports mild pain on deep palpation of the skin located just superior and medial to the port. No indication of fluid infiltration under the skin is detected. Vital signs included pulse of 95 bpm, temperature of 97.7°F (36.5°C), and blood pressure of 110/72 mm Hg.

The patient is sent urgently to interventional radiology for a fluoroscopic examination of her port. Of the 20 ml of forcefully injected contrast, approximately 1 ml was found to have extravasated at the level of the right clavicle, superior to her port (see Figure 14-2). This

Figure 14-2. Fluoroscopy of Extravasation Injury

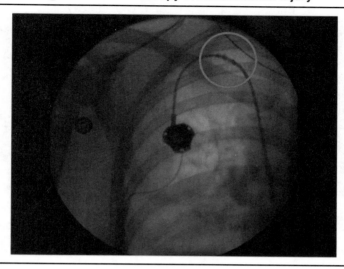

Note. Image courtesy of Daniel A. MacManus. Used with permission.

type of injury or fracture is known as pinch-off syndrome (Aitken & Minton, 1984; El Hammoumi et al., 2014; Lin et al., 2010), where scissoring or pinching of the catheter occurs between the clavicle and first rib during arm and shoulder movement. This can ultimately lead to transection and embolization of the catheter (see Figure 14-3). A dislodged intravascular catheter may be associated with pulmonary embolism, cardiac perforation, and sepsis (Wu et al., 2011). The catheter may also fracture from incorrect fixation of the catheter to the locking steel ring on the port, repeated high-pressure injections to resolve clot formation, and alteration of the catheter mechanical properties (Filippou, Tsikkinis, Filippou, Nissiotis, & Rizos, 2004).

Because it cannot be determined when the catheter became compromised, causing extravasation (two of the agents being vesicants), L.B. is referred urgently to the emergency department for initiation of antidote therapies. She is admitted overnight to receive both dexrazoxane to help treat the possibility of doxorubicin extravasation and hyaluronidase (Vitrase®) for possible vinblastine extravasation. Dexrazoxane binds to iron, preventing the formation of free radicals, which are thought to play a major role in the development of extravasation-induced tissue necrosis (Boschi & Rostagno, 2012).

Figure 14-3. Computed Tomography Scan of Catheter Embolization, Coronal and Sagittal Images

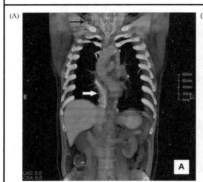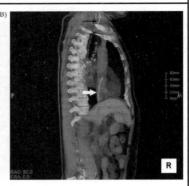

(A) coronal image; (B) sagittal image.

Note. From "Embolization of a Fractured Central Venous Catheter Placed Using the Internal Jugular Approach," by A. Shimizu, A. Lefor, M. Nakata, U. Mitsuhashi, M. Tanaka, and Y. Yasuda, 2014, *International Journal of Surgery Case Reports, 5,* p. 220. doi:10.1016/j.ijscr.2014.02.001. Copyright 2014 by Elsevier. Reprinted with permission.

Dexrazoxane is administered as an IV infusion daily for three days for anthracycline extravasation (see Table 14-2). Dexrazoxane also is used to prevent anthracycline-based cardiac toxicities.

Hyaluronidase is an enzyme that degrades hyaluronic acid, improving the absorption of extravasated drugs (Pérez Fidalgo et al., 2012). Hyaluronidase is administered as multiple subcutaneous (SC) injections (see Table 14-2) (Beaulieu, 2012; Pérez Fidalgo et al., 2012) around the periphery of the extravasation injury (see Figure 14-4). In L.B.'s case, the site to be injected was at the region of tenderness and evidence of contrast extravasation as seen on fluoroscopic evaluation.

Key Points

- Antidote therapy should be initiated without delay.
- Providers should be trained in these procedures.
- Dexrazoxane is given IV daily for three days for anthracycline extravasation.
- Hyaluronidase is given as multiple SC injections for vinca alkaloid extravasation.

Table 14-2. Vesicant Extravasation Intervention

Drug Class	Non-Drug Treatment	Suggested Drug Treatment
Alkylating agents	Cold compress applied for 6–12 hours after administration of sodium thiosulfate	Sodium thiosulfate 1/6 M (4 ml 10% sodium thiosulfate + 6 ml sterile water = 1/6 M): Instill via SC multiple injections using small-gauge needle.
Anthracyclines	Cold compress applied immediately for 20 min QID × 3 days. Remove at least 15 minutes prior to dexrazoxane treatment.	Dexrazoxane (3-day course): Administer 1,000 mg/m^2 IV within 6 hours of extravasation on day 1, 1,000 mg/m^2 on day 2, and 500 mg/m^2 on day 3.
Antitumor antibiotics	Cold compress applied immediately for 20 min QID × 3 days	No known antidotes or treatments
Platinum analogs*	Cold compress applied immediately for 20 min QID × 3 days. If using sodium thiosulfate, apply cold pack for 6–12 hours after administration of sodium thiosulfate.	Sodium thiosulfate 1/6 M (4 ml 10% sodium thiosulfate + 6 ml sterile water = 1/6 M): Instill via SC multiple injections using small-gauge needle.
Taxanes	Cold compress applied immediately for 20 min QID × 3 days	Hyaluronidase: Administer 150–1,500 units injected SC into multiple sites using small-gauge needle.
Vinca alkaloids	Warm compress applied immediately for 20 min QID × 3 days	Hyaluronidase: Administer 150–1,500 units injected SC into multiple sites using small-gauge needle.

* Have been reported as mild vesicants, depending upon concentration and amount extravasated

QID—four times a day; SC—subcutaneous

Note. Based on information from Boschi & Rostagno, 2012; Gonzalez, 2013; Pérez Fidalgo et al., 2012, Polovich et al., 2014.

From "Management of Chemotherapy Extravasations," by M. Cassagnol and A. McBride, 2009, *U.S. Pharmacist, 34*(Suppl. 9), 3–11. Retrieved from http://www.uspharmacist.com/content/s/94/c/15675. Copyright 2009 by Jobson Medical Information LLC. Adapted with permission.

Figure 14-4. Treatment Injection Sites for Hyaluronidase

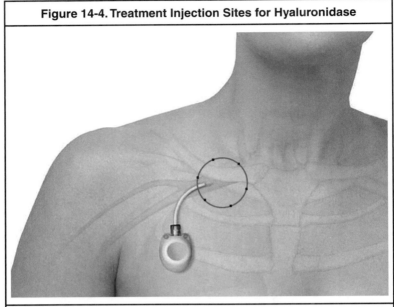

Note. From "A Brief Introduction to Ports," by Bard Access Systems, Inc. Retrieved from http://www.portadvantage.com/patient/about_implanted_ports.html. Copyright 2015 by C. R. Bard, Inc. Adapted with permission.

L.B. is discharged from the hospital after completing the first-day regimen of extravasation antidote therapy. On the second and third day, she is treated in the outpatient infusion center. This treatment includes administration of dexrazoxane IV over one to two hours, evaluation by a provider, and patient education. Dexrazoxane 1,000 mg/m² was given on days 1 and 2 and 500 mg/m² on day 3 (Schulmeister, 2011). The provider assessed for erythema, induration, ecchymosis, SC edema, warmth, discharge at each daily visit, and subsequent phone call monitoring.

What patient teaching is appropriate for this patient?

The patient is instructed about the signs and symptoms of extravasation (see Table 14-1). This discussion includes contributing factors of developing an extravasation, such as patient movement, pulling on the IV line, or problems with the port or catheter (see Table 14-3). The nurse also provides contact information in the event of an emergency and for follow-up care (e.g., plastic surgery, occupational therapy, physical therapy), should tissue integrity or mobility be compromised.

What is the pathophysiology of tissue damage?

Tissue damage depends on the chemotherapy agent's capacity to bind with DNA. DNA-binding agents cause lethal DNA cross-linking or strand breaks caused by free radicals, leading to cell death (Cheung-Ong, Giaever, & Nislow, 2013). DNA-binding agents include anthracyclines, platinum analogs, antitumor anti-

Table 14-3. Non-Medication–Related Risks for Extravasation		
Device Type	Patient-Related Risks	Clinician-Related Risks
Peripheral		

• Use of butterfly needle
• Lack of blood return
• Inadequately secured needle/catheter
• Placement in undesired location
  – Antecubital fossa
  – Dorsum of hand
  – Wrist
  – Areas of flexion/movement-prone
  – Legs or feet
• Catheter diameter/length not appropriate to size of vein
	• Age (very young or elderly)
	• Hard or sclerosed veins
	• Small veins
	• Fragile veins
	• Impaired communication or altered sensory perception
	  – Sedation/somnolence
	  – Unconscious/comatose
	• Patient movement
	  – Vomiting
	  – Seizures
	  – Coughing
	  – Stretching
	  – Lymphedema
	• Obesity
	• Multiple courses of treatment
		• Lack of IV insertion skills/education
		• Probing during insertion
		• Interruptions/distractions during administration

		(Continued on next page)

Table 14-3. Non-Medication–Related Risks for Extravasation *(Continued)*

Device Type	Patient-Related Risks	Clinician-Related Risks
Central Line		

• Huber needle misplacement or displacement to port
• Catheter separation, migration, or fracture
• Mechanical occlusion
  – Thrombus formation
  – Drug precipitate
  – Retrograde catheter displacement
  – Pinch-off
  – Fibrin sheath formation
• Port placement
  – Abdominal vascular port—increased risk for needle migration
  – Flipping of port
  – Long dwell time
  – Deeply implanted
	• Impaired communication or altered sensory perception
	• Patient movement
	• Obesity
	• Multiple courses of treatment
		• Lack of noncoring needle insertion skills/education
		• Needle length too short for depth of port access
		• Improper securing of needle device
		• Not visualizing good blood return
		• Using small-gauge syringes (e.g., 1 ml, 3 ml) for drug administration or flushing
		• Interruptions/distractions during administration

Note. Based on information from Pérez Fidalgo et al., 2012.

biotics, and some alkylating agents. Non–DNA-binding agents, such as vinca alkaloids, taxanes, and topoisomerase inhibitors, interfere with mitosis. These agents typically cause less tissue damage than DNA-binding agents (Cassagnol & McBride, 2009). Irritant drugs can cause pain at the injection site or along the vein, with or without an inflammatory reaction. Some of these agents can potentially cause soft tissue ulcers. Frequently used vesicant and irritant chemotherapy agents are highlighted in Table 14-4.

Other physiochemical factors can influence, and usually increase, the risk of extravasation injury of individual drugs. These

References

Aitken, D.R., & Minton, J.P. (1984). The "pinch-off sign": A warning of impending problems with permanent subclavian catheters. *American Journal of Surgery, 148,* 633–636. doi:10.1016/0002-9610(84)90340-4

Al-Benna, S., O'Boyle, C., & Holley, J. (2013). Extravasation injuries in adults. *ISRN Dermatology, 2013,* Article 856541. doi:10.1155/2013/856541

Beaulieu, M.J. (2012). Hyaluronidase for extravasation management. *Neonatal Network, 31,* 413–418. doi:10.1891/0730-0832.31.6.413

Biffi, R., de Braud, F., Orsi, F., Pozzi, S., Mauri, S., Goldhirsch, A., ... Andreoni, B. (1998). Totally implantable central venous access ports for long-term chemotherapy: A prospective study analyzing complications and costs of 333 devices with a minimum follow-up of 180 days. *Annals of Oncology, 9,* 767–773. doi:10.1023/A:1008392423469

Boschi, R., & Rostagno, E. (2012). Extravasation of antineoplastic agents: Prevention and treatments. *Pediatric Reports, 4,* e28. doi:10.4081/pr.2012.e28

Cassagnol, M., & McBride, A. (2009). Management of chemotherapy extravasations. *U.S. Pharmacist, 34*(Suppl. 9), 3–11. Retrieved from http://www.uspharmacist.com/content/s/94/c/15675

Cheung-Ong, K., Giaever, G., & Nislow, C. (2013). DNA-damaging agents in cancer chemotherapy: Serendipity and chemical biology. *Chemistry and Biology, 20,* 648–659. doi:10.1016/j.chembiol.2013.04.007

Clark, E., Giambra, B.K., Hingl, J., Doellman, D., Tofani, B., & Johnson, N. (2013). Reducing risk of harm from extravasation: A 3-tiered evidence-based list of pediatric peripheral intravenous infusates. *Journal of Infusion Nursing, 36,* 37–45. doi:10.1097/NAN.0b013e3182798844

Dougherty, L., & Oakley, C. (2011). Advanced practice in the management of extravasation. *Cancer Nursing Practice, 10*(5), 16–21. doi:10.7748/cnp2011.06.10.5.16.c8568

El Hammoumi, M., El Ouazni, M., Arsalane, A., El Oueriachi, F., Mansouri, H., & Kabiri, E. (2014). Incidents and complications of permanent venous central access systems: A series of 1,460 cases. *Korean Journal of Thoracic and Cardiovascular Surgery, 47,* 117–123. doi:10.5090/kjtcs.2014.47.2.117

Filippou, D.K., Tsikkinis, C., Filippou, G.K., Nissiotis, A., & Rizos, S. (2004). Rupture of totally implantable central venous access devices (intraports) in patients with cancer: Report of four cases. *World Journal of Surgical Oncology, 2,* 36. doi:10.1186/1477-7819-2-36

Gault, D.T. (1993). Extravasation injuries. *British Journal of Plastic Surgery, 46,* 91–96. doi:10.1016/0007-1226(93)90137-Z

Gonzalez, T. (2013). Chemotherapy extravasations: Prevention, identification, management, and documentation. *Clinical Journal of Oncology Nursing, 17,* 61–66. doi:10.1188/13.CJON.61-66

Goolsby, T.V., & Lombardo, F.A. (2006). Extravasation of chemotherapeutic agents: Prevention and treatment. *Seminars in Oncology, 33,* 139–143. doi:10.1053/j.seminoncol.2005.11.007

Harrold, K., Gould, D., & Drey, N. (2013). The efficacy of saline washout technique in the management of exfoliant and vesicant chemotherapy extravasation: A historical case series report. *European Journal of Cancer Care, 22,* 169–178. doi:10.1111/ecc.12023

Lin, C.H., Wu, H.S., Chan, D.C., Hsieh, C.B., Huang, M.H., & Yu, J.C. (2010). The mechanisms of failure of totally implantable central venous access system: Analysis of 73 cases with fracture of catheter. *European Journal of Surgical Oncology, 36,* 100–103. doi:10.1016/j.ejso.2009.07.011

Narducci, F., Grande, R., Mentuccia, L., Trapasso, T., Sperduti, I., Magnolfi, E., ... Gamucci, T. (2012). Symptom improvement as prognostic factor for survival in cancer patients undergoing palliative care: A pilot study. *Supportive Care in Cancer, 20,* 1221–1226. doi:10.1007/s00520-011-1207-8

Pérez Fidalgo, J.A., García Fabregat, L., Cervantes, A., Margulies, A., Vidall, C., & Roila, F. (2012). Management of chemotherapy extravasation: ESMO–EONS clinical practice guidelines. *European Journal of Oncology Nursing, 16,* 528–534. doi:10.1016/j.ejon.2012.09.004

Pikó, B., Laczó, I., Szatmári, K., Bassam, A., Szabó, Z., Ócsai, H., & Csotye, J. (2013). Overview of extravasation management and possibilities for risk reduction based on literature data. *Journal of Nursing Education and Practice, 3*(9), 93–105. doi:10.5430/jnep.v3n9p93

Polovich, M., Olsen, M., & LeFebvre, K.B. (Eds.). (2014). *Chemotherapy and biotherapy guidelines and recommendations for practice* (4th ed.). Pittsburgh, PA: Oncology Nursing Society.

Sauerland, C., Engelking, C., Wickham, R., & Corbi, D. (2006). Vesicant extravasation part I: Mechanisms, pathogenesis, and nursing care to reduce risk. *Oncology Nursing Forum, 33,* 1134–1141. doi:0.1188/06.ONF.1134-1141

Schulmeister, L. (2009). Vesicant chemotherapy extravasation antidotes and treatments. *Clinical Journal of Oncology Nursing, 13,* 395–398. doi:10.1188/09.CJON.395-398

Schulmeister, L. (2011). Extravasation management: Clinical update. *Seminars in Oncology Nursing, 27,* 82–90. doi:10.1016/j.soncn.2010.11.010

Steiert, A., Hille, U., Burke, W., Gohritz, A., Zilz, S., Herold, C., & Vogt, P.M. (2011). Subcutaneous wash-out procedure (SWOP) for the treatment of chemotherapeutic extravasations. *Journal of Plastic, Reconstructive and Aesthetic Surgery, 64,* 240–247. doi:10.1016/j.bjps.2010.04.040

Vidall, C., Roe, H., Dougherty, L., & Harrold, K. (2013). Dexrazoxane: A management option for anthracycline extravasations. *British Journal of Nursing, 22*(17), S6–S12. doi:10.12968/bjon.2013.22.Sup17.S6

Wu, C.Y., Fu, J.Y., Feng, P.H., Kao, T.C., Yu, S.Y., Li, H.J., ... Hsieh, H.C. (2011). Catheter fracture of intravenous ports and its management. *World Journal of Surgery, 35,* 2403–2410. doi:10.1007/s00268-011-1200-x

CASE 15
Myelosuppression

Barbara J. Wilson, MS, RN, AOCN®, ACNS-BC

A 66-year-old woman with ovarian cancer

S.H. is a 66-year-old woman diagnosed with stage IIIB epithelial ovarian cancer. She is a retired dental office manager and the mother of two adult daughters. Her medical history includes rheumatoid arthritis and migraine headaches. She is allergic to penicillin, noting that she developed hives when she took it as a teenager. Her current home medications include several over-the-counter nonsteroidal anti-inflammatory drugs (NSAIDs) taken as needed for headaches and arthritic pain. Her family history includes a maternal grandmother with breast cancer.

It is estimated that 21,980 new cases of ovarian cancer will be diagnosed in 2015 in the United States (American Cancer Society, 2015). In the early stages, signs and symptoms are nonspecific and not obvious until the disease advances to later stages. The most significant risk factor is a family history of breast or ovarian cancer (American Cancer Society, 2015).

S.H.'s presenting symptoms include abdominal bloating and change in bowel elimination. After an ultrasound, elevated CA-125 finding, and physical examination, she is informed of the probability of ovarian cancer. Her treatment plan includes surgery for diagnosis, staging, and cytoreduction. The treatment intent for stage IIIB ovarian cancer is to prolong survival. After surgery, adjuvant chemotherapy with paclitaxel 80 mg/m² on days 1, 8, and 15 and carboplatin AUC 6 IV every three weeks for six cycles is planned (National Comprehensive Cancer Network® [NCCN®], 2014b).

Several days after having a port placed, S.H. is scheduled for cycle 1 of chemotherapy. Her height is 68 in. (172.72 cm), and she weighs 168 lbs (76.2 kg). Her baseline complete blood count (CBC) reveals the following: White blood cell (WBC) count = 6.5×10^9 cells/L, absolute neutrophil count (ANC) = $2,100/mm^3$, platelets = $180,000/mm^3$, hemoglobin = 12.5 g/dl.

Her orders are

- Paclitaxel 80 mg/m^2 IV over one hour on days 1, 8, and 15
- Carboplatin AUC 6 IV on day 1. Repeat every three weeks for six cycles
- Famotidine 20 mg IV 30–60 minutes before paclitaxel
- Diphenhydramine 25 mg IV 30–60 minutes before paclitaxel
- Dexamethasone 10 mg IV 30 minutes before paclitaxel.

What education is essential to minimize adverse events following treatment with this regimen?

In addition to risks for hypersensitivity reactions during the treatment, myelosuppression is a concern with both paclitaxel and carboplatin and is considered a dose-limiting toxicity. More specifically, thrombocytopenia is recognized as a dose-limiting toxicity of carboplatin. Information about other side effects, including peripheral neuropathy, nausea and vomiting, alopecia, and fatigue, must also be included in the patient education (Bristol-Myers Squibb Co., 2010, 2011; Polovich, Olsen, & LeFebvre, 2014).

Key Points

- Myelosuppression is a dose-limiting toxicity of many chemotherapy agents, including paclitaxel and carboplatin.
- Myelosuppression can include neutropenia, thrombocytopenia, and anemia.

Does S.H. have any risk factors for developing febrile neutropenia?

Yes. Patient-related factors that increase the occurrence of neutropenia include age (65 years or older), gender (more prevalent in women), and recent surgery. Ovarian cancer is a disease-related risk. The carboplatin and paclitaxel regimen carries an intermediate treatment-related risk for febrile neutropenia (Irwin, Erb, Williams, Wilson, & Zitella, 2013), for which growth factor prophylaxis should be considered but is not always necessary. The physician discusses this with S.H. and decides to closely monitor her CBC during the first cycle.

How would the nurse know when a patient has febrile neutropenia?

Febrile neutropenia (FN) is a serious adverse event associated with myelosuppressive therapy. FN is defined as a single oral temperature that is greater than 38.3°C or greater than 38°C for more than one hour and either an ANC less than 500/mm^3 or an ANC less than 1,000/mm^3 that is predicted to decline to less than 500/mm^3 during the next 48 hours (NCCN, 2014c).

Before S.H.'s second cycle, her CBC results are WBC count = 3.5 × 10^9 cells/L, ANC = 1,400/mm^3, platelets = 140,000/mm^3, and hemoglobin = 11.5 g/dl. The nurse notices that values are lower than baseline but still within normal limits. S.H. reports that she feels fatigued. Vital signs are within normal limits. She receives her second cycle of chemotherapy. The patient asks the nurse if her blood counts will remain in a safe range after this treatment.

The nurse responds, "Chemotherapy can have a cumulative effect, meaning more chemotherapy may lead to an increase in side effects. You are still at risk for low blood counts after your treatment, so watching for and preventing infection and bleeding and managing fatigue will be important, as long as you are taking chemotherapy. It will also be important for you to notify our call desk any time, including nights and weekends, if you have a fever, easy bruising, or bleeding."

In addition to teaching, what should the nurse assess to ensure S.H. takes an active role in preventing and managing side effects?

The nurse should assess home medications, lifestyle, activities, and environment for potential risks. The patient should confirm that she has and knows how to use a thermometer, can state what temperature should be reported, and can describe signs and symptoms of infection, including redness and tenderness in the area of her implanted port.

S.H. arrives for her third cycle of chemotherapy. During her assessment, S.H. asks why she has a rash. The nurse notices petechiae on S.H.'s ankles. Her CBC results are WBC count = 1.5 × 10^9 cells/L, ANC 900/mm^3, platelets 65,000/mm^3, and hemoglobin = 10.4 g/dl. S.H. is informed that her blood counts are too low to safely receive therapy that day.

S.H. is anxious and wonders what can be done. The nurse should assess home medications with attention to NSAIDs used for arthritis by this patient. NSAIDs can increase bleeding risks and mask fever (Dunning & Fischbach, 2011). The nurse should emphasize hand-washing technique and frequency, the importance of monitoring for and reporting elevated temperature (greater than 38°C), and other signs of infection or bleeding, especially redness or tenderness around her port (Irwin et al., 2013).

S.H.'s chemotherapy is delayed for one week. When she arrives a week later, her WBCs, platelets, and hemoglobin have returned to normal. S.H. reports that, as recommended, she stopped taking the NSAIDs because she is concerned about their effect on her platelet count and masking fever. Instead, she is using nonpharmacologic interventions that have helped her in the past. The nurse notes a new order for filgrastim, a granulocyte–colony-stimulating factor (G-CSF), beginning on day 2 of this cycle and discusses this with S.H. (NCCN, 2014a).

What patient education should be provided to S.H. before administering the granulocyte–colony-stimulating factor?

In addition to the benefits of G-CSFs in reducing the time to neutrophil recovery between treatments and decreasing the duration of neutropenia, side effects should be explained. Bone pain related to increased growth of myeloid cells over a short period of time in the bone marrow may be a concern. Because S.H. already has rheumatoid arthritis, additional bone pain may require more or different pain management interventions.

S.H. has been listening to other patients in the treatment center talk about low blood counts and asks the nurse if she can eat salads and fresh fruits.

How should the nurse answer this question?

The nurse provides a teaching handout and reviews the evidence-based information for prevention of infection. Based on recent studies, when patients have neutropenia, they should avoid eating foods that are not washed or cooked. For example, eating fresh fruits that have been washed is acceptable practice, but eating raw eggs or raw meat is not recommended (Irwin et al., 2013; Polovich et al., 2014).

S.H. receives filgrastim following cycles 4 and 5. She experiences a dose reduction of her chemotherapy drugs with cycle 5 for platelet count 92,000/mm^3. When she arrives for her sixth and last cycle, her CBC results are WBC = 3.4 × 10^9 cells/L, ANC = 2,000/mm^3, platelets = 95,000/mm^3, and hemoglobin = 10.1 g/dl. She has no symptoms of bleeding, bruising, or petechiae. When discussing options with her physician, S.H. chooses a dose delay over dose reduction for her sixth cycle so she can travel to a family wedding that she would not have been able to attend if she had treatment that week.

Conclusion

While S.H. was receiving myelosuppressive chemotherapy, she experienced dose delays and dose reductions. The treatment intent was not curative, so maintaining quality of life and minimizing side effects are appropriate goals during therapy. A number of risk factors for neutropenia and thrombocytopenia contributed to the occurrence and severity of these side effects. Because assessments and interventions were timely, neutropenia did not lead to febrile neutropenia, and the thrombocytopenia resulted in petechiae without either occult or overt bleeding. She did not receive prophylactic G-CSF before her first two cycles of chemotherapy based on risk assessment; however, she required G-CSF therapy following cycles 3–5 because of dose-limiting neutropenia (WBC = 1.5 × 10^9 cells/L) (NCCN, 2014a).

References

American Cancer Society. (2015). *Cancer facts and figures 2015*. Retrieved from http://www.cancer.org/research/cancerfactsstatistics/cancerfactsfigures2015/index.

Bristol-Myers Squibb Co. (2010). *Paraplatin® (carboplatin)* [Package insert]. Princeton, NJ: Author.

Bristol- Myers Squibb Co. (2011). *Taxol® (paclitaxel)* [Package insert]. Princeton, NJ: Author.

Dunning, M.B., & Fischbach, F. (2011). *Common laboratory and diagnostic tests* (5th ed.). Philadelphia, PA: Lippincott Williams & Wilkins.

Irwin, M.M., Erb, C., Williams, C., Wilson, B.J., & Zitella, L.J. (2013). *Putting evidence into practice: Improving oncology patient outcomes—Prevention of infection*. Pittsburgh, PA: Oncology Nursing Society.

National Comprehensive Cancer Network. (2014a). *NCCN Clinical Practice Guidelines in Oncology (NCCN Guidelines®): Myeloid growth factors* [v.2.2014]. Retrieved from http://www.nccn.org/professionals/physician_gls/pdf/myeloid_growth.pdf

National Comprehensive Cancer Network. (2014b). *NCCN Clinical Practice Guidelines in Oncology (NCCN Guidelines®): Ovarian cancer including fallopian tube cancer and primary peritoneal cancer* [v.1.2015]. Retrieved from http://www.nccn.org/professionals/physician_gls/pdf/ovarian.pdf

National Comprehensive Cancer Network. (2014c). *NCCN Clinical Practice Guidelines in Oncology (NCCN Guidelines®): Prevention and treatment of cancer-related infections* [v.2.2014]. Retrieved from http://www.nccn.org/professionals/physician_gls/pdf/infections.pdf

Polovich, M., Olsen, M., & LeFebvre, K.B. (Eds.). (2014). *Chemotherapy and biotherapy guidelines and recommendations for practice* (4th ed.). Pittsburgh, PA: Oncology Nursing Society.

CASE 16
Nausea and Vomiting

Kathy Mooney, MSN, APRN-CNS, OCN®, BMTCN™

A 36-year-old woman with lymphoma

J.C. is a 36-year-old woman with a history of relapsed diffuse large cell lymphoma who achieved a complete remission after eight cycles of R-CHOP (rituximab, cyclophosphamide, doxorubicin, vincristine, and prednisone). J.C. has a past surgical history of tonsillectomy. She denies alcohol use, smoking, or illicit substance use.

She is currently admitted for a myeloablative matched related bone marrow transplant using the following preparative regimen:
- Busulfan 1 mg/kg PO on days −6 through −3
- Cyclophosphamide 50 mg/kg IV on days −2 and −1
- Cyclophosphamide 50 mg/kg IV on days +3 and +4 for graft-versus-host disease prophylaxis.

Prior to beginning chemotherapy regimens, what should the nurse understand about the emetogenic potential of different chemotherapy regimens?

Chemotherapy agents and regimens are classified according to emetic risk as highly emetogenic, moderately emetogenic, low emetogenic, and minimally emetogenic. Of patients who receive highly emetogenic regimens, 90% have emesis if not treated with prophylactic antiemetics. This rate decreases to 30% with the use of antiemetics prior to treatment (National Comprehensive Cancer Network® [NCCN®], 2014). Antiemetic guidelines use these classifications to make recommendations to prevent or minimize nausea and/or vomiting. According to NCCN, the best practice is to begin antiemetic ther-

141

apy prior to the first dose of chemotherapy and to continue as long as the chemotherapy agent has the potential to cause nausea or vomiting.

Oral busulfan has a moderate risk for emesis; therefore, J.C. is given ondansetron 16 mg PO prior to the first dose and then every 24 hours through day −4 of her preparative regimen. Because cyclophosphamide is considered highly emetogenic, patients are treated with combination antiemetic therapy, started prior to the first dose of chemotherapy. J.C.'s antiemetic regimen for her cyclophosphamide is as follows:

- Serotonin (5-HT$_3$) antagonist: Ondansetron 8 g IV every 12 hours for 8 doses
- Steroid: Dexamethasone 10 mg IV every 24 hours for 2 doses (only used for cyclophosphamide given prior to transplant)
- Neurokinin-1 receptor antagonist: Fosaprepitant 150 mg IV once
- Antianxiety agent: Lorazepam 0.5 mg IV every 24 hours for two doses.

What other information should the RN obtain related to nausea and vomiting before beginning chemotherapy regimens?

The RN should assess the patient for prior tolerance of chemotherapy agents and be aware of any history of nausea and vomiting. Chemotherapy-induced nausea and vomiting (CINV) can be classified as acute, delayed, anticipatory, or breakthrough (NCCN, 2014). Acute-onset CINV occurs within minutes to hours after the chemotherapy infusion and will usually resolve within 24 hours. Delayed-onset CINV begins more than 24 hours after the chemotherapy infusion and can last for days following the infusion. Delayed-onset CINV commonly occurs with cisplatin, carboplatin, cyclophosphamide, and doxorubicin. Anticipatory CINV occurs before patients receive their chemotherapy infusion as a conditioned response to a previous negative experience with chemotherapy. Breakthrough CINV occurs despite the use of prophylactic antiemetics and requires the use of additional antiemetic drugs (NCCN, 2014). Other risk factors for increased CINV include bowel obstruction, brain metastases, electrolyte imbalances, gastroparesis, uremia, anxiety, anticipatory nausea/vomiting, history of motion sickness, female gender, and younger age (NCCN, 2014).

J.C. has multiple risk factors for increased CINV. She reports a history of nausea with her R-CHOP regimen, as well as a history of motion sickness. She is also a young woman, which further increases her risk.

What patient teaching should the nurse include prior to beginning chemotherapy regimens?

Patients should be educated about the potential for nausea and vomiting with each chemotherapy administration. They should be aware of the antiemetic regimen prescribed and the availability of treatment for breakthrough occurrences. Patients should be instructed that eating small, frequent meals; avoiding greasy, fried, salty, sweet, or spicy foods; and eating food at room temperature may help to control nausea and vomiting (National Cancer Institute, 2012).

On day −3 to transplant, J.C. begins experiencing nausea. She receives lorazepam 0.5 mg IV PRN with good relief. By day 0, the PRN lorazepam is not controlling her nausea, and J.C. begins receiving PRN ondansetron 8 mg IV in addition to lorazepam. On day 4, after receiving her post-transplant cyclophosphamide, J.C.'s nausea is not controlled, and she is now having episodes of emesis as well.

How is breakthrough nausea best managed?

When nausea is not controlled, it is considered best practice to add an additional agent from a different class of drugs to control nausea and vomiting. It is also considered best practice to schedule antiemetics around the clock rather than use a PRN schedule to control nausea and vomiting (NCCN, 2014). Patients who are experiencing vomiting should be given IV medications instead of oral medications. It may be necessary to administer multiple antiemetics on an alternating schedule to gain control of nausea and vomiting (NCCN, 2014).

After speaking with the patient about the available antiemetics and her previous response to them, J.C.'s oncology team decides to schedule ondansetron 8 mg IV every eight hours. J.C. also continues to receive PRN doses of lorazepam. After three days on this regimen, J.C.'s nausea and vomiting worsens, and it is decided to add scheduled lorazepam 0.5 mg IV every six hours to her antiemetic regimen.

What consequences of nausea and vomiting should the RN be aware of when caring for patients?

It is important for the RN to assess patients' abilities to take oral medications, maintain adequate oral intake, and monitor for electrolyte abnormalities (NCCN, 2014). Patients who have uncontrolled nausea and vomiting may need to have their medications switched to the IV route for a period of time. Patients who experience uncontrolled nausea and vomiting are at a greater risk for malnutrition, which may increase morbidity, mortality, infections, pressure ulcers, and falls (Davidson et al., 2012). The nurse should monitor for signs and symptoms of electrolyte imbalances and dehydration. This includes tracking the patient's weight, noting the patient's intake and output, and monitoring laboratory results (Bender et al., 2002).

What nonpharmacologic strategies are available for chemotherapy-induced nausea and vomiting?

Hypnosis, progressive muscle relaxation, guided imagery, and managing patient expectations are considered likely to be effective in reducing or preventing CINV. Other nonpharmacologic strategies have not been established as effective in reducing CINV (Lee et al., 2014). Oncology nurses should offer patients information about these nonpharmacologic techniques when appropriate.

J.C.'s nausea is better controlled after scheduling around-the-clock antiemetics, and she has no further episodes of emesis. After two additional days of this regimen and with her nausea controlled, J.C. requests to try PRN antiemetics instead of a scheduled regimen. It is decided to change her lorazepam to PRN and continue the scheduled ondansetron for 24 hours to monitor any change in her nausea. After 24 hours, J.C. continues to feel well, and her ondansetron is also changed to PRN.

Key Points

- The best practice is to begin antiemetic therapy prior to the first dose of chemotherapy and to continue as long as the chemotherapy agent has the potential to cause nausea or vomiting (NCCN, 2014).
- CINV can be classified as acute, delayed, anticipatory, or breakthrough (NCCN, 2014).
- When nausea is not controlled, it is considered best practice to add an additional agent from a different class of drugs to try to control nausea and vomiting (NCCN, 2014).

- Patients who experience uncontrolled nausea and vomiting are at a greater risk for malnutrition, which may increase morbidity, mortality, infections, pressure ulcers, and falls (Davidson et al., 2012).

Conclusion

Despite pharmacologic advances, CINV is a potential significant side effect of chemotherapy that continues to affect patients. Chemotherapy agents and regimens are classified according to emetic risk, and antiemetic guidelines use these classifications to make recommendations to prevent or minimize nausea and vomiting. Oncology nurses should be aware of the emetic potential of the chemotherapy they are administering, as well as the patient's risk factors and previous experiences with CINV. The RN should ensure that patients have received education regarding CINV, including prevention strategies and treatment regimens.

References

Bender, C.M., McDaniel, R.W., Murphy-Ende, K., Pickett, M., Rittenberg, C.N., Rogers, M.P., … Schwartz, R.N. (2002). Chemotherapy-induced nausea and vomiting. *Clinical Journal of Oncology Nursing, 6,* 94–102. doi:10.1188/02.CJON.94-102

Davidson, W., Teleni, L., Muller, J., Ferguson, M., McCarthy, A.L., Vick, J., & Isenring, E. (2012). Malnutrition and chemotherapy-induced nausea and vomiting: Implications for practice [Online exclusive]. *Oncology Nursing Forum, 39,* E340–E345. doi:10.1188/12.ONF.E340-E345

Lee, J., Cherwin, C., Czaplewski, L.M., Dabbour, R., Doumit, M., Duran, B., … Whiteside, S. (2014). Putting evidence into practice: Chemotherapy-induced nausea and vomiting. Retrieved from https://www.ons.org/practice-resources/pep/chemotherapy-induced-nausea-and-vomiting

National Cancer Institute. (2012). Managing chemotherapy side effects. Nausea and vomiting. Retrieved from http://www.cancer.gov/publications/patient-education/nausea.pdf

National Comprehensive Cancer Network. (2014). *NCCN Clinical Practice Guidelines in Oncology (NCCN Guidelines®): Antiemesis* [v.2.2014]. Retrieved from http://www.nccn.org/professionals/physician_gls/PDF/antiemesis.pdf

Renal Toxicity

Barbara J. Wilson, MS, RN, AOCN®, ACNS-BC

A 61-year-old man with small cell lung cancer

E.G. is a 61-year-old man with a 40-pack-year history of smoking and recent onset of persistent productive cough. He is referred to the multidisciplinary lung clinic by his primary care physician when a 4.2 cm mass in the right upper lobe is seen on a computed tomography (CT) scan of his chest. His workup includes a positron-emission tomography (PET) scan, magnetic resonance imaging scan of the brain, complete blood count (CBC), and chemistry profile. He is also scheduled for a bronchoscopy and a follow-up appointment to the clinic.

During his next appointment, E.G. is informed that he has extensive-stage small cell lung cancer (SCLC) involving his right lung, liver, ribs, sternum, bilateral scapula, humeri, and brain. SCLC is staged as limited or extensive, which is different from other solid tumor staging that uses the tumor-node-metastasis (TNM) staging classification (National Comprehensive Cancer Network® [NCCN®], 2015).

Laboratory results reveal CBC, blood urea nitrogen (BUN), creatinine, and electrolytes all within normal limits, except for a serum calcium of 10.9 mg/dl that is slightly above normal range of 8.4–10.3 mg/dl (Dunning & Fischbach, 2011).

The nurse reviews E.G.'s medical history of acute viral hepatitis in the distant past, multiple hip and pelvic fractures sustained in a motorcycle accident, nephrolithiasis, and recently diagnosed enlarged prostate. His wife has been with him for all tests and appointments, and he reports that he is employed full time as a construction contractor.

At this time, he is 5'9" (180 cm) and weighs 191 lbs (86.6 kg); despite the extent of his disease, he appears healthy. E.G. denies pain, weight loss, hemoptysis, dyspnea, and cognitive changes. Vital signs are recorded as blood pressure of 123/71 mm Hg, heart rate of 95 bpm, temperature of 96.2°F (35.6°C), respiratory rate of 16 breaths per min, and pulse oximetry of 98% on room air.

Based on cell type and extent of disease, his treatment plan is for cranial irradiation and chemotherapy with cisplatin 60 mg/m² and etoposide 120 mg/m² on days 1–3 every 21 days for six cycles (NCCN, 2015).

Within a week, E.G. has a port inserted, attends a class with his wife that will help prepare him for chemotherapy, and is scheduled for his first treatment with the following orders:
• IV 1,000 ml normal saline (NS) with 20 mEq potassium chloride at 500 ml/hr
• Aprepitant 125 mg PO on day 1 and 80 mg PO on days 2 and 3
• Palonosetron 0.25 mg IV on day 1
• Dexamethasone 12 mg PO on day 1 and 8 mg PO on days 2–4
• Cisplatin 60 mg/m² IV in 500 ml NS over 60 minutes on day 1
• Etoposide 120 mg/m² IV days 1–3 in 500 ml NS over 60 minutes
• Zoledronic acid 4 mg IV over 15 minutes every four weeks.

Side effects of cisplatin, such as nausea, vomiting, nephrotoxicity, and peripheral neuropathy, should be included in the chemotherapy teaching. Severe chemotherapy-induced nausea and vomiting (CINV), both acute and delayed, are associated with the alkylating agent cisplatin. Nephrotoxicity can be a dose-limiting side effect of cisplatin and the risk for acute kidney injury can increase as the cumulative dose increases. Peripheral neuropathy is common with cisplatin and also worsens as the cumulative dose increases. Diarrhea, mucositis, and photosensitivity are common side effects of antimetabolite chemotherapy (Polovich, Olsen, & LeFebvre, 2014), but not cisplatin.

E.G. states that he has difficulty voiding and prefers to defer large amounts of fluid until he gets home from work to avoid frequent trips to the restroom when at his work site. He also shares that in the past when he has been ill and nauseated, he avoids eating and drinking until the feeling subsides. This is not safe because even though E.G. has started his chemotherapy, acute and delayed nausea and vomiting can lead to dehydration.

Dehydration, in addition to cisplatin therapy, may increase the risk for renal toxicity. Adequate oral intake and voiding at regular intervals are essential to monitoring and maintaining adequate renal function (Felver, 2013; Polovich et al., 2014).

Key Points
- Controlling nausea and vomiting as a result of cisplatin therapy is essential to prevent dehydration.
- Dehydration, in addition to recent therapy with cisplatin, may increase the risk for renal toxicity.

Teaching strategies at the chemotherapy class have been effective for E.G. and his wife. E.G. states he understands the importance of reporting if he experiences concentrated urine, decreased urinary output, or inability to maintain oral intake for any reason. He verbalizes understanding that blood tests will be done to assess his kidney function prior to each cycle and that he will receive IV fluids before each treatment. In addition, E.G.'s wife states that she understands from the information presented that it is important for E.G. to prevent kidney damage by drinking plenty of fluids.

Asking patients and significant others to summarize key points of teaching is one way to evaluate teaching effectiveness. Asking open-ended questions creates an opportunity for the nurse to validate accurate information and to correct any misunderstandings the patient or significant other may have.

Because E.G. has extensive bone metastases, he is at risk for skeletal complications (Brant, 2014). His treatment plan includes a bone-targeting bisphosphonate drug called zoledronic acid, which is prescribed every four weeks with evaluation of renal function and serum calcium before each dose (Novartis Pharmaceuticals Corp., 2014). Before his third dose of zoledronic acid, the nurse notices that his BUN is 21 mg/dl and serum creatinine is 1.3 mg/dl, both slightly above the upper limit of normal. Although his serum calcium is now 10.1 mg/dl, which is decreased from baseline but within normal limits, why should the nurse be concerned? Zoledronic acid can adversely affect renal function and should be withheld for renal deterioration.

The physician discontinues the zoledronic acid and orders a receptor activator of nuclear factor-κB (known as RANK) ligand inhibitor called denosumab, which does not require dose adjustments for renal function but can also cause hypocalcemia (Amgen Inc., 2014).

During cycles 1–3 of cisplatin and etoposide, E.G. is compliant with instructions for hydration, antiemetics, and willingness to report any problems or symptoms at onset. He has minimal nausea, and his appetite, voiding, and weight are without change. After cycle 3, a PET-CT scan is done, demonstrating partial response with a decrease in the size of the lung, bone, and liver lesions. The physician uses Response Evaluation Criteria In Solid Tumors (known as RECIST) criteria (version 1.1) for partial response defined as 30% reduction in the sum of diameters of target lesions compared to the baseline (Polovich et al., 2014). E.G. is scheduled to receive three more cycles. He has been feeling well and is back to working a limited schedule (half days in the morning). After his fourth treatment and the good news about his treatment response, he is less diligent about oral hydration and taking antiemetics. During the three days following his fourth treatment, E.G. experiences nausea but avoids vomiting by not eating or drinking. E.G. becomes weak, and his wife recognizes signs of dehydration and calls the clinic. When E.G. is assessed, his weight has decreased to 182 lbs (82.5 kg), his skin turgor is poor, and he appears weak and tired. Blood tests reveal elevated BUN of 25 mg/dl and serum creatinine of 2.7 mg/dl. His vital signs are blood pressure of 96/60 mm Hg, heart rate of 92 bpm, and temperature of 97.2°F (36.2°C).

What would E.G. benefit from most at this time?

He should receive IV fluids for immediate rehydration and IV antiemetics, as oral intake is not feasible for him at this time. The nurse should be aware that side effects of cisplatin and etoposide do not decrease with subsequent treatments. Interviewing the patient about side effect management and asking for "teach back" will ensure that education has been effective.

Conclusion

Because of timely and accurate assessments of his renal function, E.G. completed all six cycles of chemotherapy without dose delays or reductions. Awareness that his chemotherapy regimen, bone-targeting medications, and lifestyle could affect renal function was appropriately included in assessments. The nurse plays an active role in ensuring that laboratory parameters for renal function are monitored and reported to the physician and that the patient and family are involved in assessing and reporting side effects.

References

Amgen Inc. (2014). *Xgeva® (denosumab)* [Package insert]. Thousand Oaks, CA: Author.

Brant, J.M. (2014). Pain. In C.H. Yarbro, D. Wujcik, & B.H. Gobel (Eds.), *Cancer symptom management* (4th ed., pp. 67–89). Burlington, MA: Jones & Bartlett Learning.

Dunning, M.B., & Fischbach, F. (2011). *Nurses' quick reference to common laboratory and diagnostic tests* (5th ed.). Philadelphia, PA: Wolters Kluwer Health/Lippincott Williams & Wilkins.

Felver, K. (2013). Fluid, electrolyte, and acid-base balance. In P.A. Potter, A.G. Perry, P.A. Stockert, & A.M. Hall (Eds.), *Fundamentals of nursing* (8th ed., pp. 882–939). St. Louis, MO: Elsevier Mosby.

National Comprehensive Cancer Network. (2015). *NCCN Clinical Practice Guidelines in Oncology (NCCN Guidelines®): Small cell lung cancer* [v.1.2015]. Retrieved from http://www.nccn.org/professionals/physician_gls/pdf/sclc.pdf

Novartis Pharmaceuticals Corp. (2014). *Zometa® (zoledronic acid)* [Package insert]. East Hanover, NJ: Author.

Polovich, M., Olsen, M., & LeFebvre, K.B. (Eds.). (2014). *Chemotherapy and biotherapy guidelines and recommendations for practice* (4th ed.). Pittsburgh, PA: Oncology Nursing Society.

CASE 18
Cardiotoxicity

Lisa S. Moss, ANP-C, MSN, AOCNP®

A 44-year-old woman with hormone receptor–positive breast cancer

M.Z. is a 44-year-old woman with right-sided stage IIIA (pT3N2MX), estrogen receptor–positive, progesterone receptor–positive, HER2/neu-positive breast cancer, diagnosed after a self-palpated mass. M.Z. is premenopausal prior to administration of chemotherapy. Her past medical history includes hypertension, hyperlipidemia, and obesity (body mass index of 38.5).

Preoperative imaging includes a computed tomography scan of the chest, abdomen, and pelvis as well as a bone scan, which are both negative for any metastatic disease; and magnetic resonance imaging scan of the breast, which is negative for any contralateral disease in the left breast.

M.Z. undergoes surgery that involves a right modified radical mastectomy and left prophylactic mastectomy. The postoperative treatment includes

- Doxorubicin and cyclophosphamide IV every three weeks for four cycles
- Paclitaxel and trastuzumab IV weekly for 12 weeks, followed by trastuzumab for a total of one year
- Initiation of endocrine therapy.

What findings would increase M.Z.'s risk for cardiotoxicity?

Cardiotoxicity is an alteration in cardiac function. Cardiac events can differ based on the medication administered. M.Z.'s regimen includes doxorubicin and trastuzumab, both of which carry the risk of cardiotoxicity; the risk increases when the patient receives both agents.

When reviewing a patient's history, particularly if he or she is receiving a cardiotoxic medication, it is important to assess other risk factors for heart disease. According to the National Heart, Lung, and Blood Institute (2014), risk factors for heart disease include high blood pressure, high cholesterol, diabetes, smoking, being overweight or obese, physical inactivity, family history of heart disease, and unhealthy diet.

Based on the data provided, the nurse knows M.Z. will have an increased risk because she is receiving two medications with the potential for cardiotoxicity. Other relevant risk factors include her personal history of hypertension, hyperlipidemia, and obesity.

Some risk factors for heart disease, such as family history, are not modifiable. Others, such as hypertension, hyperlipidemia, diet, activity level, and obesity, can be modified. When conducting a risk assessment for patients receiving cardiotoxic medications, the nurse must identify modifiable risk factors and educate the patients about a proactive approach to decreasing the risk of heart damage by working on these factors. For example, M.Z. can coordinate visits with her primary care provider to ensure her hypertension and hyperlipidemia are well controlled, work with a dietitian or obtain resources with regard to a healthy diet, and develop an individualized plan for increased physical activity. In addition, when the healthcare team recognizes a patient who has multiple risk factors, such as M.Z., they can plan increased monitoring for signs and symptoms related to cardiotoxicity.

Key Points

- All patients should undergo a cardiotoxicity risk assessment when receiving doxorubicin and/or trastuzumab.
- Patients with multiple risk factors should be monitored more closely during cardiotoxic chemotherapy.

After completion of doxorubicin, an echocardiogram (echo) is done, with a reported ejection fraction of 60%. Repeat echo three months after initiation of trastuzumab shows an ejection fraction of 55%. Six months after initiation of trastuzumab, the ejection fraction is 42%.

What symptoms and physical examination findings would the nurse assess to determine if M.Z.'s decreased ejection fraction is symptomatic or asymptomatic?

Patients may present with a decreased ejection fraction and have no symptoms at all. Conversely, patients may have complaints or particular findings on physical examination that classify them as "symptomatic." In addition to laboratory and diagnostic tests, subjective data and objective findings are important. Prior to administration of each cycle of treatment, a review of systems and physical examination should be performed to determine if the patient has any signs of heart damage. Specific objective findings include the following symptoms: shortness of breath or dyspnea, fatigue, weight gain, swelling in extremities, or a nonproductive cough. Objective signs indicating cardiotoxicity can include tachycardia or arrhythmias, jugular vein distention, hypotension, lower extremity edema, and an S3 or S4 heart sound or murmur (Walker, 2015). Positive findings may require further evaluation.

Key Points
- Patients receiving cardiotoxic medications should have cardiac testing at baseline and periodically during their treatments.
- Positive physical findings should be reported to the provider prior to administration of treatment.

Based on an assessment of her symptoms, it is determined that M.Z. has an asymptomatic decline in her ejection fraction. An order is written to resume trastuzumab and follow up with repeat echocardiogram in three months. Is this an appropriate order?

The trastuzumab package insert addresses the potential for cardiotoxicity and makes recommendations for monitoring and adjustments in treatment based on findings. With regard to cardiac testing, left ventricular ejection fraction (LVEF) should be evaluated prior to and at regular intervals during treatment. There is no specification regarding the interval timing of testing or what type of test to perform (e.g., echo versus multigated acquisition scan).

Guidelines have been developed to address a decline in LVEF regardless of whether the patient is symptomatic or asymptomatic. Trastuzumab should be withheld for four weeks if a patient has a decline in LVEF of 16% or greater or if the LVEF is below the institutional limits of normal and greater than or equal to a 10% decrease from pretreatment testing. If the LVEF returns to normal and the absolute decrease from baseline is less than or equal to 15% from baseline, treatment can be resumed.

M.Z. has a drop in her LVEF by more than 16%; therefore, her treatment should be withheld for four weeks—when LVEF will be reassessed—regardless of her symptoms.

Oncology nurses have a professional responsibility to be familiar with recommendations regarding oncology treatment and advocate on behalf of patients. Bringing such information to the attention of a provider may spare the patient further cardiac damage and complications. This is important with all patients being treated with curative intent, but particularly with young patients like M.Z. With continued advancements in oncology treatment, nurses have the potential to cure more patients; however, patients could be left with lifelong complications such as cardiotoxicity.

Key Point

- Oncology nurses must have knowledge of guidelines regarding managing patients with decreased LVEF.

What are the recommendations for cardiac surveillance following administration of trastuzumab in the adjuvant setting?

M.Z. is seen for routine evaluation two years after completion of treatment and remains on endocrine therapy. Based on recommendations from Genentech outlined in the package insert, patients treated with trastuzumab in the adjuvant setting should undergo evaluation of LVEF every six months for two years after completion of therapy (Genentech, Inc., 2014). Many patients are seen following completion of adjuvant therapy in survivorship clinics and receive a post-treatment summary and plan of care. This information is shared with the patient and others involved in the objective of care. The potential for cardiotoxicity and the need for ongoing monitoring are areas that should be addressed during these visits. Healthcare providers can work collaboratively to determine who will be responsible for cardiac monitoring after completion of therapy.

Conclusion

Cancer is diagnosed in patients of all age groups and with varying levels of comorbid conditions. Treatment regimens are often complex, with multiple drugs having additive toxicity. Oncology nurses play a key role in educating patients about potential side effects and reportable conditions. With education and careful monitoring, complications from treatment can be decreased, leading to improved patient outcomes.

References

Genentech, Inc. (2014). *Herceptin® (trastuzumab)* [Package insert]. South San Francisco, CA: Author.

National Heart, Lung, and Blood Institute. (2014). What are the risk factors for heart disease? Retrieved from http://www.nhlbi.nih.gov/health/educational/hearttruth/lower-risk/risk-factors.htm

Walker, D.K. (2015). Alterations in cardiovascular function. In J.K. Itano (Ed.), *Core curriculum for oncology nursing* (5th ed., pp. 393–403). St. Louis, MO: Elsevier.

CASE 19
Reproductive Toxicity

Marjorie Weiman, RN, MSN, CPHON®

A 23-year-old woman with Ewing sarcoma

T.K. is a 23-year-old woman with pain in her right thigh and knee. She attributes this pain to an aggressive exercise regimen that she has just started, and the pain seems to go away with rest. However, the pain continues and progresses in intensity, and five months later she sees an orthopedic surgeon. Plain x-rays are normal, and she is diagnosed with patellar tendinitis. T.K. is given a brace and nonsteroidal anti-inflammatory drugs and is shown some stretching exercises. Despite these measures, her pain increases; she has a magnetic resonance imaging (MRI) scan two months later. The MRI shows a very large lesion (10 cm in length) in her right femur and an associated soft tissue mass. An open biopsy is done and reveals Ewing sarcoma. Her metastatic workup is negative.

By the time of her diagnosis, T.K. is in excruciating pain and requires high doses of opioids. Possible side effects are discussed with the patient and her parents prior to beginning chemotherapy. Loss of fertility is discussed, and fertility preservation options are briefly addressed, but the patient opts to not pursue any options at the time. She tells her mother that she is so overwhelmed by both the diagnosis and the amount of pain that she cannot possibly consider anything other than treatment of her disease.

What contributes to the loss of fertility in patients with cancer?

Many factors contribute to the development of infertility in patients with cancer, and it is safe to say that no two patients have the same risk.

Some general risk factors for both men and women are older age at diagnosis, ovarian/uterine or hypothalamic/pituitary radiation, surgical removal of a gonad, and treatment with alkylating agents or bleomycin sulfate (Green et al., 2009; Wasilewski-Masker et al., 2014). Table 19-1 reviews the potential for infertility with several chemotherapeutic agents.

When should loss of fertility be addressed with patients?

The American Society of Clinical Oncology recommends that shortly after diagnosis, all patients should receive information about potential loss of fertility. Fertility preservation options should also be made available to children and adolescents in conjunction with their parents (Loren et al., 2013). Patients report being reassured by receiving this information, as it seems to impart that their treating physician believes they will survive their cancer and it gives them hope for the future at a very bleak moment in their lives.

Table 19-1. Chemotherapeutic Agents Associated With Infertility Risks

Risk Level	Agents
High	• Cyclophosphamide • Busulfan • Chlorambucil • Procarbazine • Melphalan • Ifosfamide • Mechlorethamine
Medium	• Cisplatin and carboplatin • Doxorubicin • Docetaxel • Paclitaxel
Low	• Vincristine and vinblastine • Bleomycin • Methotrexate • Fluorouracil • Mercaptopurine

Note. Based on information from Blumenfeld, 2012.

What options are available to patients who decide they want children?

Survivors are now more vocal about wanting to know their options if they are interested in becoming parents, and clinicians realize that fertility options need to be introduced to patients immediately after diagnosis (Loren et al., 2013). However, the options for men and women differ greatly in both ease and cost. For postpubertal boys and men, semen cryopreservation is the gold standard for fertility preservation. Cancer survivors have a few options available to them, including adoption, although some states in the United States and some countries do not allow cancer survivors to adopt children (Gardino, Russell, & Woodruff, 2010). Some agencies, however, are very welcoming to cancer survivors, stating that birth mothers have known someone with cancer and do not seem concerned about prospective parents with a history of cancer. Other options available to female patients, depending on their circumstances and their reproductive specialists, include harvesting and cryopreserving the survivor's eggs; using egg donors, in which the survivor carries the baby to full term; or seeking surrogates who can carry the pregnancy while using either donated eggs or the survivor's eggs.

How long does it take to harvest eggs if done prior to chemotherapy?

Many clinicians are concerned about the length of time that it might take to harvest eggs and the resultant delay in treatment. In the past, ovarian stimulation occurred in synchronization with the patient's menstrual cycle, and there could often be a delay of four to six weeks. However, it is becoming more common to start the ovarian stimulation protocol immediately after patient presentation without waiting for menstrual cycle synchronization, resulting in a delay of only two to three weeks (Cakmak & Rosen, 2013).

What should be cryopreserved: Oocytes or embryos?

In the past, only embryo cryopreservation was offered. Women who had partners or who wanted to use donor sperm could exercise this option. Since October 2012, the American Society for Reproductive Medicine no longer considers oocyte cryopreservation experimental, and the success rate for live births from cryopreserved oocytes is similar to the rate for freshly harvested eggs (Oktay, Cil, & Bang, 2006). All postpubertal girls and women now have the potential option of storing oocytes for in vitro fertilization and implantation.

T.K. receives standard chemotherapy for treatment of Ewing sarcoma, consisting of alternating cycles of vincristine, doxorubicin, and cyclophosphamide with ifosfamide and etoposide. She also receives surgery for local control with a total replacement of her femur after 12 weeks of chemotherapy. During treatment, she has prolonged periods of neutropenia and admissions for pain control and nutrition issues related to mucositis. She finally completes nine months of therapy, and surveillance scans continue to show no evidence of disease.

What is the risk of infertility with alkylating agents?

Clinicians often struggle with knowing that chemotherapy can cause infertility but not being able to quantify the risk for certain chemotherapy regimens. Studies measure the accumulated dose of alkylating agents (AAD) by assigning cumulative doses of agents to a tertile and assigning a number to each tertile (1 [lowest tertile], 2 [middle tertile], and 3 [highest tertile]). For example, T.K.'s chemotherapy regimen placed her AAD score at 6. Any regimen with an AAD score higher than 3 or 4 results in patients being less likely to become pregnant (Green et al., 2009). More recently, Green et al. (2014) have demonstrated a formula for calculating a cyclophosphamide equivalent dose in order to compare doses across regimens.

What effect does chemotherapy have on the number of eggs available?

Women are born with the entire number of oocytes they will ever have. The number of oocytes decreases with age, and the loss accelerates after age 37.5 (Faddy, Gosden, Gougeon, Richardson, & Nelson, 1992). When the number of oocytes falls to around a thousand, menopause ensues (see Figure 19-1). When a woman receives chemotherapy or radiation, the oocytes can become injured in the process, and the total number of oocytes available to a woman for future fertility decreases. Patients who have been treated for cancer can enter menopause at a younger age than untreated cohorts. In years past, after treatment for cancer, women were urged not to delay pregnancies, as premature menopause was a significant concern.

During one of her post-treatment visits to the clinic, T.K. asks her physician if she would need to use birth control if she was having sexual intercourse. T.K. says that she thinks she might be infertile because of the cancer treatment and does not need to worry about birth control. The physician explains that T.K. does need to use birth control measures if she does not want to become pregnant.

How is the resumption of menses correlated with fertility?

It is not. Many studies assume that resumption of menses is a marker for fertility and that amenorrhea is a marker for infertility. But in 1990, it was shown that in patients who had been treated for breast cancer, pregnancies occurred in women who were not menstruating (Sutton, Buzdar, & Hortobagyi, 1990). In women who are

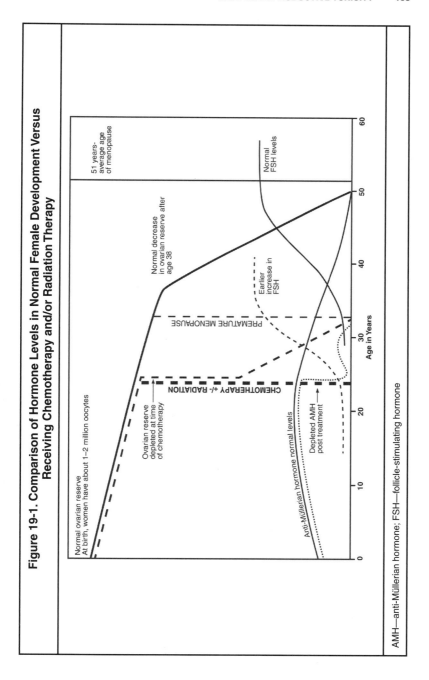

Figure 19-1. Comparison of Hormone Levels in Normal Female Development Versus Receiving Chemotherapy and/or Radiation Therapy

AMH—anti-Müllerian hormone; FSH—follicle-stimulating hormone

menstruating following treatment, lower levels of ovarian reserve have also been found (Larsen, Müller, Schmiegelow, Rechnitzer, & Andersen, 2003).

Approximately six months after completion of treatment, T.K. asks her physician about whether she could get pregnant. She has a boyfriend with whom she is considering marriage, and she wants to know what her options are regarding the possibility of children. She knew there was a possibility she could have problems having children but is unsure if this is still true. The physician explains that, given all the chemotherapy she received, it is likely that T.K. is sterile, and he refers her to a reproductive specialist for further counseling. The reproductive specialist who sees T.K. draws an anti-Müllerian hormone (AMH) level, carefully reviews her chart for her chemotherapy history, and sits down with T.K. for a lengthy consultation.

How does anti-Müllerian hormone level help predict fertility?

AMH has been recognized as a marker for ovarian reserve that does not fluctuate with the menstrual cycle. The molecule is decreased in patients who are no longer fertile and absent in patients in menopause. Anderson, Rosendahl, Kelsey, and Cameron (2013) recommended drawing a level prior to treatment in order to estimate a woman's eventual risk for infertility based on both AMH and age at diagnosis. An AMH level greater than 2 ng/ml prior to chemotherapy will result in a faster recovery of AMH level after treatment. Women who start with lower AMH levels have much slower recovery of AMH, which can be an indicator that women who are less fertile going into treatment are at higher risk for becoming completely infertile after treatment (Dillon et al., 2013).

The reproductive specialist explains to T.K. that her AMH level and her exposure to very high amounts of alkylating agents for her cancer treatment have left her at a very high risk for infertility. Her AMH level is 0.9 ng/ml. T.K. becomes distraught at the thought of not being able to be a biological mother and requests an attempt to harvest and freeze oocytes. The reproductive specialist agrees to attempt ovarian stimulation. She is started on the protein hormone gonadotropin as part of a conventional ovarian stimulation protocol. At the appropriate time of the cycle, a transvaginal approach is used to harvest mature oocytes, but unfortunately, no viable specimens are found. Because each of these procedures can cost \$6,000–\$10,000, T.K. cannot afford further stimulation and harvesting attempts at this time. The cost of the drugs and the procedure are not covered by her insurance. Although disappointed, T.K. decides not to pursue further reproductive technologies at this time.

Key Points

- Fertility preservation should be offered to all newly diagnosed patients with cancer if clinically feasible.
- If not medically contraindicated, women can harvest and store either oocytes or embryos.
- Men can cryopreserve sperm for later use.
- Chemotherapy and radiation can reduce the number of viable oocytes, especially abdominal radiation and alkylating agents.
- Female patients with cancer can enter menopause earlier as a result of treatment.
- Fertility procedures often are not covered by insurance.
- There are several pathways to parenthood that patients with cancer can take, including in vitro fertilization, using donated oocytes or sperm, surrogacy, or adoption.

Conclusion

Many new and exciting changes in fertility preservation have occurred in the past few years. The emergence of AMH as a marker for ovarian reserve with predictive value both before and after treatment is a major milestone. In addition, the ability to freeze oocytes instead of embryos for women without partners provides women with choices where there used to be none. Reproductive specialists can assist patients with post-treatment oocyte freezing to prolong fertility options, even if they were unable to harvest oocytes prior to chemotherapy. Recently, work has been ongoing to develop an immunomodulator, AS101, which shows potential as a protector of ovarian function by reducing follicle activation (Kalich-Philosoph et al., 2013). Although challenges still remain, including the cost of fertility preservation in women and lack of insurance coverage for fertility procedures, women have more choices and opportunities than ever before.

References

Anderson, R.A., Rosendahl, M., Kelsey, T.W., & Cameron, D.A. (2013). Pretreatment anti-Müllerian hormone predicts for loss of ovarian function after chemotherapy for early breast cancer. *European Journal of Cancer, 49,* 3404–3411. Retrieved from http://www.ncbi.nlm.nih.gov/pmc/articles/PMC3807650

Blumenfeld, Z. (2012). Chemotherapy and fertility. *Best Practice and Research Clinical Obstetrics and Gynaecology, 26,* 379–390. doi:10.1016/j.bpobgyn.2011.11.008

Cakmak, H., & Rosen, M.P. (2013). Ovarian stimulation in cancer patients. *Fertility and Sterility, 99,* 1476–1484. doi:10.1016/j.fertnstert.2013.03.029

Dillon, K.E., Sammel, M.D., Prewitt, M., Ginsberg, J.P., Walker, D., Mersereau, J.E., ... Gracia, C.R. (2013). Pretreatment antimüllerian hormone levels determine rate of posttherapy ovarian reserve recovery: Acute changes in ovarian reserve during and after chemotherapy. *Fertility and Sterility, 99,* 477–483.e1. doi:10.1016/j .fertnstert.2012.09.039

Faddy, M.J., Gosden, R.G., Gougeon, A., Richardson, S.J., & Nelson, J.F. (1992). Accelerated disappearance of ovarian follicles in mid-life: Implications for forecasting menopause. *Human Reproduction, 7,* 1342–1346.

Gardino, S.L., Russell, A.E., & Woodruff, T.K. (2010). Adoption after cancer: Adoption agency attitudes and perspectives on the potential to parent post-cancer. In T.K. Woodruff, L. Zoloth, L. Campo-Engelstein, & S. Rodriguez (Eds.), *Cancer Treatment and Research: Vol. 156. Oncofertility: Ethical, legal, social, and medical perspectives* (pp. 153–170). doi:10.1007/978-1-4419-6518-9_11

Green, D.M., Kawashima, T., Stovall, M., Leisenring, W., Sklar, C.A., Mertens, A.C., ... Robison, L.L. (2009). Fertility of woman survivors of childhood cancer: A report from the Childhood Cancer Survivor Study. *Journal of Clinical Oncology, 27,* 2677–2685. doi:10.1200/JCO.2008.20.1541

Green, D.M., Nolan, V.G., Goodman, P.J., Whitton, J.A., Srivastava, D., Leisenring, W., ... Robison, L.L. (2014). The cyclophosphamide equivalent dose as an approach for quantifying alkylating agent exposure: A report from the Childhood Cancer Survivor Study. *Pediatric Blood and Cancer, 61,* 53–67. doi:10.1002/pbc.24679

Kalich-Philosoph, L., Roness, H., Carmely, A., Fishel-Bartal, M., Ligumsky, H., Paglin, S., ... Meirow, D. (2013). Cyclophosphamide triggers follicle activation and "burnout"; AS101 prevents follicle loss and preserves fertility. *Science Translational Medicine, 5,* 185ra62. doi:10.1126/scitranslmed.3005402

Larsen, E.C., Müller, J., Schmiegelow, K., Rechnitzer, C., & Andersen, A.N. (2003). Reduced ovarian function in long-term survivors of radiation- and chemotherapy-treated childhood cancer. *Journal of Clinical Endocrinology and Metabolism, 88,* 5307–5314. doi:10.1210/jc.2003-030352

Loren, A.W., Mangu, P.B., Beck, L.N., Brennan, L., Magdalinski, A.J., Partridge, A.H., ... Oktay, K. (2013). Fertility preservation for patients with cancer: American Society of Clinical Oncology clinical practice guideline update. *Journal of Clinical Oncology, 31,* 2500–2510. doi:10.1200/JCO.2013.49.2678

Oktay, K., Cil, A.P., & Bang, H. (2006). Efficiency of oocyte cryopreservation: A meta-analysis. *Fertility and Sterility, 86,* 70–80. doi:10.1016/j.fertnstert.2006.03.017

Sutton, R., Buzdar, A.U., & Hortobagyi, G.N. (1990). Pregnancy and offspring after adjuvant chemotherapy in breast cancer patients. *Cancer, 65,* 847–850.

Wasilewski-Masker, K., Seidel, K.D., Leisenring, W., Mertens, A.C., Shnorhavorian, M., Ritenour, C.W., … Meacham, L.R. (2014). Male infertility in long-term survivors of pediatric cancer: A report from the Childhood Cancer Survivor Study. *Journal of Cancer Survivorship, 8,* 437–447. doi:10.1007/s11764-014-0354-6

Survivorship Care Planning

Syndal Ortman, APRN, DNP, FNP-BC

A 50-year-old man with tongue cancer

R.W. is a 50-year-old man with a history of stage IVA (T2, N2, M0) tongue cancer diagnosed more than four years ago after presenting to his primary care provider with right neck pain, dysphagia, and a mass on his tongue for three weeks. He underwent a right modified neck dissection levels 1–3 followed by chemotherapy with six cycles of carboplatin and paclitaxel, as well as radiation to the tongue and upper and lower neck areas. He had been lost to follow-up with all of his healthcare providers for more than a year and now presents with persistent headaches, pain in his shoulders and neck, dry mouth, extreme fatigue, dysphagia, and depression.

What should first be assessed when seeing a cancer survivor with new symptoms?

The first priority is to rule out recurrence or a secondary malignancy. Subjectively, R.W. says he has not had any fevers, chills, or weight loss. He has severe fatigue that may be aggravated by trouble sleeping at night from neck and shoulder pain as well as an inability to find a comfortable lying position. He has not noticed any cognitive changes or memory loss. He has a poor appetite and eats mostly soft foods as a result of his dysphagia. He does not have any throat or mouth pain and has not noticed any new masses or lumps. He denies any hearing changes or tinnitus. His skin has been dry without rashes, but he reports persistent itching around his neck. He denies cough, chest pain, palpitations, or shortness of breath. He is not having any numbness, tingling, or pain in his hands or feet. He is depressed, mostly because he feels he is disabled. He used to enjoy his work as a cook but is now unable to even make a meal for himself at home. His adult son comes over to help him with daily activities such as dressing, cooking, and cleaning. R.W. is embarrassed to ask his son to help him in the shower, so he will do what he can by himself, even if it causes more pain. He does not drive because he is unable to turn his head from side to side, so he uses public transportation. He does not exercise like he used to because of his fatigue and pain. He says he feels hopeless being in pain all the time and does not see how his quality of life could ever improve. He does not talk to his family or friends about his chronic issues since completing cancer treatments because they all think he should be happy to have survived cancer and do not understand why he has withdrawn from family and social events. He is divorced and was in a long-term relationship that ended while he was going through chemotherapy. He would like companionship but believes his physical ailments and disabilities prevent him from ever being in a physical or emotional relationship again. He is not currently sexually active and has erectile dysfunction. He is always concerned that his cancer might return, which is why he has avoided his follow-up appointments until now.

R.W.'s physical examination reveals decreased range of motion in his right shoulder, scapular winging posture, and inability to turn his head to the right or left because of pain and stiffness. He has sharp, shooting pain down his spine with forward flexion of the head. No lesions, masses, or redness in the mouth or tongue are detected, and his buccal mucosa appears dry. His right neck area shows postsurgical changes and radiation-induced mildly hyperpigmented skin. No palpable cervical, supraclavicular, axillary, or inguinal lymphadenopathy is detected. The thyroid is symmetric without nodules, lung sounds are clear to auscultation bilaterally in all fields, and heart sounds have regular rate and rhythm without murmurs. Laboratory tests at this visit include a complete blood count, comprehensive metabolic panel, and thyroid-stimulating hormone (TSH) (see Table 20-1).

What late or long-term side effects are associated with cancer treatment?

Each cancer survivor's experience with treatment is unique, and the patient should be educated on the potential late and long-term side effects that may result from surgery, chemotherapy, and radiation therapy. Knowledge of each treatment received by the cancer survivor is important in order to identify potential late or long-term

Table 20-1. R.W.'s Laboratory Test Results

Test	Reference Range	Result
Thyroid-stimulating hormone	0.3–4.2 mU/L	11.4 mU/L
Hemoglobin	13.1–17.5 g/dl	17.2 g/dl
Platelets	150–400 K/mm^3	186 K/mm^3
White blood cells	4.0–10 K/mm^3	5.1 K/mm^3
Glucose	70–100 mg/dl	100 mg/dl
Sodium	135–148 mEq/L	142 mEq/L
Potassium	3.5–5.3 mEq/L	4.2 mEq/L
Chloride	100–108 mEq/L	103 mEq/L
Carbon dioxide	22–30 mEq/L	30 mEq/L
Blood urea nitrogen	6–20 mg/dl	11 mg/dl
Creatinine	0.70–1.2 mg/dl	0.8 mg/dl
GFR, African American	No range found	132 ml/min
GFR, non–African American	No range found	109 ml/min
Anion gap	7–14 mEq/L	9 mEq/L
Calcium	8.6–10 mg/dl	9.8 mg/dl
Albumin	3.4–5 g/dl	4.8 g/dl
Total protein	6.4–8.3 g/dl	7.5 g/dl

GFR—glomerular filtration rate

Note. Reference ranges are based on those used at Hennepin County Medical Center.

side effects and intervene early. According to Hewitt, Greenfield, and Stovall (2006), late effects of cancer treatment are side effects that are "absent or subclinical at the end of therapy and become manifest later" (p. 69), possibly months or even years after treatment has been completed. Long-term side effects "refer to any side effects or complications of treatment" that would manifest itself during treatment and persists after treatment has completed (Hewitt et al., 2006, p. 69).

Carboplatin has been associated with a risk for ototoxicity and peripheral neuropathy (Lee & Wen 2014b), and paclitaxel also increases R.W.'s risk for peripheral neuropathy (Lee & Wen, 2014a). Paclitaxel may damage the sensory nerve fibers or cause a motor neuropathy, most commonly in the hands or feet. This side effect is often dose-dependent, and the risk increases when given with other potentially neurotoxic agents such as other platinum chemotherapies. Chemotherapy also poses other potential complications such as bone marrow suppression, myelodysplastic syndrome, and other secondary blood disorders (e.g., leukemia) (Cancer.net, 2014).

A lifelong change in vocal ability and swallowing function may result from head and neck cancer treatment (Limaye & Haddad, 2012). Survivors may have a negative body image or self-image as a result. With speech difficulty, they may become socially isolated and avoid seeing family and friends or returning to work. A persistent difficulty with swallowing makes social gatherings a place of anxiety for head and neck cancer survivors who may be physically unable to swallow food by mouth or have trouble controlling their secretions and also increases their risk for aspiration. With many social and family gatherings or holidays revolving around eating and drinking, cancer survivors might decide to avoid these situations out of embarrassment or depression. Neck stiffness and pain also are common and may be associated with fibrosis or lymphedema (Hutcheson & Lewis, 2014).

What risks do cancer survivors face after receiving radiation to the chest and neck? What should be monitored?

It is important to be aware of the areas in which a patient receives radiation therapy because it introduces the risk for skin changes or skin cancer in the radiation field, secondary malignancies, or dysfunction of the underlying organs or tissues (American Cancer Society, 2014).

Radiation to the oral cavity can cause permanent damage to salivary glands, resulting in xerostomia, or dry mouth syndrome (Limaye & Haddad, 2012). Chronic dry mouth can be very uncomfortable for patients, with limited treatment options. This puts patients at an increased risk for dental caries and osteoradionecrosis, or bone death, of the jaw. Thickened secretions, along with dysphagia, may lead to aspiration and infection in head and neck cancer survivors. Radiation treatment may also be associated with trismus or other temporomandibular joint dysfunction, causing chronic pain, headaches, or difficulty eating. Radiation to the neck can cause thyroid dysfunction (Dubner, 2013), and TSH should be monitored every 6–12 months and as clinically indicated. Another complication also associated with neck radiation is carotid artery stenosis, which can lead to an increased risk of stroke (Saba & Leem, 2014).

What prevention measures and other screenings are appropriate?

It is evaluated whether R.W. has need for other cancer screenings. He has no family history of colon cancer and has never had a colonoscopy. However, R.W. is eligible for colorectal cancer screening (CRC) because the recommended age for beginning CRC screenings is 50 (National Comprehensive Cancer Network®, 2014). He is a nonsmoker and not at an increased risk for lung cancer. It is important to note that this also decreases his risk for tongue cancer recurrence (Brockstein, Stenson, & Song, 2014). He has not seen his primary care provider for a health maintenance examination in more than three years.

What diagnoses would the nurse identify for R.W.?

- Long-term effects of treatment
  - R.W. is experiencing chronic pain syndrome, secondary to neck dissection, radiation fibrosis, and possible Lhermitte sign (Lim et al., 2010). Pain and stiffness began after surgery and have worsened and persisted over time. This is a long-term effect of his cancer treatments.
  - Xerostomia and dysphagia began during treatments and persisted over time, so they are also long-term effects.
- Late side effects of treatment
  - Thyroid dysfunction, as a result of radiation to the neck, is diagnosed years after he completed his radiation; this is a late effect of his treatments.
  - Other late effects experienced by R.W. are depression and anxiety, secondary to disability, chronic pain, and fear of cancer recurrence.
  - R.W. is also experiencing fatigue, possibly secondary to elevated TSH and hypothyroidism.

How should R.W.'s care be coordinated?

R.W. has been lost to follow-up for some time and will need interdisciplinary referral for the management of late and long-term side effects of his cancer treatment (see Figure 20-1). The survivorship care provider will need to help R.W. navigate the healthcare system and meet his new healthcare team. His treatment summary is created, and he is counseled on follow-up guidelines and management of late and long-term side effects. Other members of the healthcare team, including the primary care provider, are given the treatment summary as well to improve coordination and responsibility of care.

Key Points

- It is important to know each treatment received by the cancer survivor in order to identify and possibly prevent potential late or long-term side effects.
- The area in which a patient receives radiation therapy is important to note because it introduces the risk for skin changes or skin cancer in the radiation field, secondary malignancies, or dysfunction of the underlying organs or tissues.
- Carotid artery stenosis is one complication associated with neck radiation, which can introduce the increased risk of stroke.
- Radiation treatment is also associated with trismus or other temporomandibular joint dysfunction and thyroid dysfunction.

Conclusion

The survivorship phase of the cancer continuum is based on recommendations in *From Cancer Patient to Cancer Survivor: Lost in Transition* (Hewitt et al., 2006). This report was released as a call to action to coordinate care for cancer survivors, improve quality of life, assess late and long-term side effects, and address the long-term needs of cancer survivors after the completion of treatment. Hewitt et al. (2006) recommended four components of survivorship care: prevention, surveillance, intervention, and coordination. Figure 20-2 illustrates the components of survivorship care, using R.W. as an exemplar.

Figure 20-1. Interdisciplinary Referral for the Management of Late and Long-Term Side Effects of Cancer Treatment

- Referral to pain specialist to evaluate options to manage chronic pain and muscle stiffness
- Referral to ear, nose, and throat specialists for a surveillance exam and possible flexible laryngoscopy to further rule out any cancer recurrence
- Referral to speech-language pathologist to evaluate dysphagia
- Referral to dentist for hygiene and checkup. Patient should have visits every six months for history of radiation and xerostomia.
- Referral to psycho-oncologist for depression and anxiety. A prescription for an antidepressant may be indicated at this visit along with discussion of strategies to manage fear of cancer recurrence, disability, and role changes.
- Referral to endocrinologist for elevated thyroid-stimulating hormone associated with fatigue, dry skin, and depression
- Referral to occupational therapist to evaluate scapular winging, chronic neck and shoulder pain, ability to perform activities of daily living, and adaptive equipment needs
- Reestablishment of primary care to address health maintenance issues such as colonoscopy, lipid panel screening, and prostate cancer screening

---

Figure 20-2. Components of Survivorship Care

Prevention

- This will include other cancer screenings and assessment for tongue cancer recurrence in collaboration with ear, nose, and throat specialist.
- Health promotion is essential to decrease the risk of future malignancies, including smoking cessation, a healthy diet, and regular exercise.
- National Comprehensive Cancer Network® guidelines for survivorship care also include a survivorship screening, which should be assessed at each clinic visit. Survivorship issues to be assessed include anxiety and depression, cognitive function, fatigue, pain, sexual function, sleep disorder, exercise, immunization, and infections.

Surveillance

- Assessment and management for cancer recurrence or metastases through history and physical exam as recommended through follow-up guidelines.
- Assessment and management of R.W.'s thyroid dysfunction, depression, chronic pain, dysphagia, and fatigue. This will also include surveillance for other potential late effects at each visit such as monitoring for osteoradionecrosis of the jaw, lymphedema, skin changes in the field of radiation, psychosocial concerns, and issues returning to work.

(Continued on next page)

Figure 20-2. Components of Survivorship Care *(Continued)*

Intervention
- This will include a multidisciplinary team to evaluate and treat R.W.'s late and long-term side effects.

Coordination
- The survivorship care provider will discuss R.W.'s treatment summary and care plan with his primary care provider and other specialists, as needed, to collaborate care. The survivorship care provider will also help coordinate these appointments and educate the patient on which providers and specialists should be seen for which issues.

Note. Based on information from Hewitt et al., 2006; National Comprehensive Cancer Network®, 2015.

Although R.W. completed his cancer treatments several years ago, he had been lost in the healthcare system for follow-up among clinical providers. Like many cancer survivors, R.W. did not know he needed routine screenings or that the effects of surgery, chemotherapy, or radiation could be managed. Attention to the physical and psychosocial side effects of cancer and its treatments, along with the coordination of care among R.W.'s healthcare team, can help to improve his quality of life, facilitate recovery to a more functional status, and improve his long-term outcomes.

References

American Cancer Society. (2014). Second cancers in adults. Retrieved from http://www.cancer.org/acs/groups/cid/documents/webcontent/002043-pdf.pdf
Brockstein, B.E., Stenson, K.M., & Song, S. (2014). Overview of treatment for head and neck cancer [UpToDate]. Retrieved from http://www.uptodate.com/contents/overview-of-treatment-for-head-and-neck-cancer
Cancer.net. (2014). Long-term side effects of cancer treatment. Retrieved from http://www.cancer.net/survivorship/long-term-side-effects-cancer-treatment
Dubner, S. (2013, August 1). Head and neck cancer—Resection and neck dissection treatment and management. Retrieved from http://emedicine.medscape.com/article/1289474-treatment#a1128
Hewitt, M., Greenfield, S., & Stovall, E. (Eds.). (2006). *From cancer patient to cancer survivor: Lost in transition.* Washington, DC: National Academies Press.
Hutcheson, K.A., & Lewis, C.M. (2014). Head and neck cancer survivorship management. In L.E. Foxhall & M.A. Rodriguez (Eds.), *Advances in cancer survivorship management* (pp. 145–166). Houston, TX: Springer.

Lee, E.Q., & Wen, P.Y. (2014a). Overview of neurologic complications of non-platinum cancer chemotherapy [UpToDate]. Retrieved from http://www.uptodate .com/contents/overview-of-neurologic-complications-of-non-platinum-cancer -chemotherapy

Lee, E.Q., & Wen, P.Y. (2014b). Overview of neurologic complications of platinum-based chemotherapy [UpToDate]. Retrieved from http://www.uptodate .com/contents/overview-of-neurologic-complications-of-platinum-based -chemotherapy

Lim, D.C., Gagnon, P.J., Meranvil, S., Kaurin, D., Lipp, L., & Holland, J.M. (2010). Lhermitte's sign developing after IMRT for head and neck cancer. *International Journal of Otolaryngology, 2010,* Article 907960. doi:10.1155/2010/907960

Limaye, S., & Haddad, R. (2012). Head and neck cancer survivorship. In K.D. Miller (Ed.), *Excellent care for cancer survivors: A guide to fully meet their needs in medical offices and in the community* (pp. 264–282). Santa Barbara, CA: Praeger.

National Comprehensive Cancer Network. (2014). *NCCN Clinical Practice Guidelines in Oncology (NCCN Guidelines®): Colorectal cancer screening* [v.1.2014]. Retrieved from http://www.nccn.org/professionals/physician_gls/pdf/colorectal_screening .pdf

National Comprehensive Cancer Network. (2015). *NCCN Clinical Practice Guidelines in Oncology (NCCN Guidelines®): Survivorship* [v.1.2015]. Retrieved from http://www .nccn.org/professionals/physician_gls/pdf/survivorship.pdf

Saba, N.F., & Leem, T. (2014). Post-treatment surveillance of squamous cell carcinoma of the head and neck [UpToDate]. Retrieved from http://www.uptodate .com/contents/posttreatment-surveillance-of-squamous-cell-carcinoma-of-the -head-and-neck?source=see_link

CASE 21
Care of a Patient Receiving a Complicated Regimen

Paula M. Muehlbauer, RN, MSN, AOCNS®

A 64-year-old man with acute lymphocytic leukemia

J.B. is a 64-year-old man who presents to his primary care provider complaining of decreased appetite, fatigue, shortness of breath, and light-headedness over the past three weeks. His physician notes a hemoglobin drop from 16.9 to 9.5 g/dl and a white blood cell (WBC) count decreased from 7,400 to 1,200/mm³ as compared to the previous year. He denies fever, chills, night sweats, easy bruising, or unusual bleeding. His skin color is pale. He has no palpable nodes or enlarged spleen on physical examination. He undergoes a bone marrow biopsy, which shows 30% blasts, consistent with acute leukemia. His diagnosis is Philadelphia chromosome–negative, acute B-cell lymphocytic leukemia. J.B. is admitted to the oncology inpatient unit to receive packed red blood cells and to start chemotherapy for acute lymphocytic leukemia (ALL).

What are specific characteristics of acute lymphocytic leukemia, and how will the nurse explain this to the patient?

Leukemia is cancer in which the bone marrow produces abnormal WBCs as a result of a defect in the stem cell. ALL is characterized by the presence of too many lymphoblasts (immature, ineffective WBCs) or too many lymphocytes in both the bone marrow and peripheral blood. ALL can spread to the lymph nodes, spleen, liver, central nervous system, and other

179

organs. Without treatment, ALL usually progresses quickly (Kurtin, 2011).

According to the American Cancer Society (2015), 6,250 new cases and 1,450 deaths from ALL were estimated for 2015. The National Cancer Institute (2014) estimates that overall survival for ALL is 66.4% in people of all ages and 90.8% in children younger than age five.

Risk factors for ALL in adults are unknown but may include prior hematologic disorder, genetic abnormalities, chemical exposures, ionizing radiation, previous cancer treatments, and autoimmune diseases (Handy, Olsen, & Zitella, 2013; Kurtin, 2011). J.B.'s history reveals extensive work with paint products and related cleaning agents and solvents.

J.B.'s symptoms are typical of presenting symptoms, except he did not experience fever, night sweats, or weight loss. Patients report signs and symptoms caused by neutropenia, thrombocytopenia, and anemia, which are related to the bone marrow infiltration with leukemic cells. Others may include cough, bone pain, headache, and lumps caused by swollen lymph nodes in and around the neck, underarm, stomach, or groin (Handy et al., 2013; Kurtin, 2011).

The treatment plan for J.B. is chemotherapy using the hyper-CVAD regimen. This regimen consists of two parts that alternate every 21 days. The first part includes cyclophosphamide, vincristine, doxorubicin, and dexamethasone. The second part includes high-dose methotrexate with leucovorin rescue, high-dose cytarabine, and methylprednisolone.

J.B.'s laboratory values on admission prior to chemotherapy are listed in Table 21-1.

What is tumor lysis syndrome?

Tumor lysis syndrome (TLS) is a syndrome of metabolic and electrolyte imbalance that occurs when rapidly growing tumors are treated with chemotherapy. Cells die and lyse, releasing intracellular electrolytes (potassium and phosphorus) and uric acid into the bloodstream. Electrolyte abnormalities associated with TLS are listed in Table 21-2. Calcium phosphate precipitates and urate crystals can form in renal tubules and ducts, sometimes resulting in renal insufficiency and failure (Polovich, Olsen, & LeFebvre, 2014; Shelton, 2009b).

Those at high risk for TLS are patients with chemotherapy-sensitive malignancies (e.g., leukemias, lymphomas, small cell lung can-

Table 21-1. Pretreatment Laboratory Values, Part 1

Test	Laboratory Value
White blood cell count	17,600/mm^3 (high)
Red blood cell count	2.90 million/mm^3 (low)
Hemoglobin	9.4 g/dl (low)
Hematocrit	28.4% (low)
Platelets	395,000/mm^3
Segmented neutrophils	43% (low)
Bands	0%
Absolute neutrophil count	7,568/mm^3
Sodium	137 mEq/L
Potassium	4.3 mEq/L
Chloride	104 mEq/L
Carbon dioxide, total	26 mEq/L
Blood urea nitrogen	14 mg/dl
Glucose	97 mg/dl
Calcium	8.6 mg/dl
Phosphate	3.3 mg/dl
Albumin	3.4 g/dl
Lactate dehydrogenase	213 U/L

Table 21-2. Laboratory Values Indicative of Tumor Lysis Syndrome

Abnormal Laboratory Result	Laboratory Value
Hyperkalemia	> 5.5 mEq/L or > 25% increase from baseline
Hyperphosphatemia	> 4.5 mg/dl or > 25% increase from baseline
Hyperuricemia	> 8 mg/dl or 25% increase from baseline
Hypocalcemia	< 7 mg/dl or 25% decrease from baseline

cer) and a high tumor burden, like J.B., and a lactate dehydroge-
nase (LDH) level greater than 1,500 mg/dl. TLS may occur in other
cancers, including melanoma, breast cancer, rhabdomyosarcoma,
and sarcoma (Shelton, 2009b).

How will the interdisciplinary team manage this patient?

- Administer vigorous hydration before, during, and after chemotherapy to maintain urine flow and prevent renal damage.
- Consider diuretics to sustain output if hydration is not sufficient.
- Administer allopurinol or rasburicase to decrease uric acid.
- Maintain alkaline urine (pH 7–7.5) to reduce the formation of
  uric acid crystals.
- Evaluate cardiac, neurologic, gastrointestinal, and renal function
  (e.g., pulse, electrocardiogram, muscle strength, laboratory values) (Shelton, 2009b).

J.B.'s oncologist orders IV hydration with 0.9% normal saline
at 150 ml/hr to maintain a euvolemic state and diuretics if
needed. Other orders include an echocardiogram; peripherally
inserted central catheter; strict intake and output; daily weights;
allopurinol 600 mg orally on day 1, then 300 mg daily; and daily
complete blood count with differential and laboratories, including potassium, uric acid, calcium, LDH, phosphate, and magne-
sium. The essential treatment goals are to prevent hyperuricemia
and hyperphosphatemia that could cause renal failure and to
prevent hyperkalemia or hypocalcemia that could cause cardiac
abnormalities.

Chemotherapy orders (based on body surface area [BSA] of
2.08) for J.B. include

- Cyclophosphamide (300 mg/m^2) 624 mg IV every 12 hours over
  3 hours on days 1–3
- Mesna (600 mg/m^2) 1,248 mg IV every day to run continu-
  ously on days 1–3, starting with the first dose of cyclophospha-
  mide
- Vincristine 2 mg IV on days 4 and 11
- Doxorubicin (50 mg/m^2) 104 mg IV on day 4
- Dexamethasone 40 mg PO every morning on days 1–4 and days
  11–14
- Filgrastim 480 mcg subcutaneous (SC) on days 5–11
- Supportive medications for nausea and vomiting.

What will the nurse teach the patient and his family about potential side effects of doxorubicin, vincristine, and cyclophosphamide?

J.B. will receive antiemetics to prevent nausea and vomiting and will be informed that doxorubicin may turn his urine red. He will be told that he may experience peripheral neuropathy from vincristine. In addition, the nurse will teach J.B. to maintain hand hygiene and perform frequent oral care to prevent infection; to increase oral fluid intake to decrease risk of hemorrhagic cystitis; to avoid sick children and large crowds or to wear a mask in public; and to take his temperature daily and immediately report fever of 100.4°F (38°C) or greater. In addition to fever, other signs and symptoms of infection include chills, sore throat, shortness of breath, pain or burning while urinating, diarrhea, mouth sores, abdominal discomfort or pain, and rectal discomfort (Wilson et al., 2014; Zitella, 2014). See Table 21-3 for a summary of patient education.

J.B. tolerates his therapy well and is discharged on day 5. He returns on day 21 for the second part of his hyper-CVAD regimen. He is alert and oriented. The nurse assesses for the following: numbness and tingling of extremities, paresthesia, dysesthesias, foot drop, and motor weakness. The nurse observes the patient's ability to button his shirt and pick up a small object and observes his gait and balance (Polovich et al., 2014). His assessment is negative for peripheral neuropathy, and he denies pain.

The nurse assesses J.B. for constipation, oral mucositis, nausea, and vomiting. J.B. reports having daily bowel movements, which are normal for him; his oral cavity looks healthy; and he denies oral pain. He has not had any nausea or vomiting since his discharge.

His vital signs are heart rate 72 beats per min; blood pressure 124/74 mm Hg; respiratory rate 16 breaths per min; temperature 98.6°F; and oxygen saturation 100% on room air.

A bone marrow biopsy indicates remission. See Table 21-4 for J.B.'s values prior to the second part of the hyper-CVAD regimen.

In addition to supportive medications for nausea and vomiting, J.B.'s chemotherapy (based on BSA 2.04) orders include

- Methylprednisolone 50 mg IV piggyback (IVPB) over 30 minutes twice daily on days 1–3
- Methotrexate (200 mg/m^2) 408 mg IVPB over two hours on day 1
- Methotrexate (800 mg/m^2) 1,632 mg IV on day 1 over 24 hours immediately after methotrexate two-hour bolus

Table 21-3. Patient Education for Part 1 of Hyper-CVAD Regimen

Chemotherapy	Side Effects	Immediate Patient Education	Discharge Patient Education
Doxorubicin	• Myelosuppression • Nausea and vomiting • Alopecia • Mucositis • May turn urine red (drug is red in color) • Dose-limiting cardiotoxicity • Radiation recall • Cardiac arrhythmia • Hyperuricemia • Photosensitivity	• Nausea and vomiting – Medicate for nausea and vomiting around the clock. – Instruct patient to eat small, frequent meals and avoid strong odors. – Help the patient to use guided imagery and progressive muscle relaxation. • Mucositis – Treat with cryotherapy. – Instruct patient to use sodium bicarbonate mouthwash after eating. – Encourage proper brushing and flossing. – Initiate institution-specific oral care protocols. • Myelosuppression – Stress importance of daily hygiene, especially hand and oral hygiene.	• Alopecia – Hair loss begins 1–3 weeks after drug administration. – Hair loss also can include eyebrows, eyelashes, and other body hair. – Patients can be given referral for wig. – Artificial eyebrows and eyelashes are available commercially; use with caution on sensitive skin. – Need to wear hat and sunscreen with sun protection factor of 15 or higher. – Patients should be reassured that hair will regrow once all alopecia-inducing treatment has ended. • Myelosuppression – Understand importance of hand hygiene, daily baths, and good oral hygiene. – Avoid crowds or wear mask in crowds. – Avoid sick children. – Take all antifungals and antibiotics if ordered.

(Continued on next page)

Table 21-3. Patient Education for Part 1 of Hyper-CVAD Regimen *(Continued)*

Chemotherapy	Side Effects	Immediate Patient Education	Discharge Patient Education
Doxorubicin *(cont.)*		– Place patient on bleeding precautions if platelet count < 100,000/mm^3	– Avoid contact with fresh flowers and plants and stagnant water. – Take temperature daily; report fever ≥ 100.4°F (38°C) and go to emergency department. • Cardiotoxicity – May be late effect of doxorubicin – Keep all records of medication administration. – Report shortness of breath or swelling of extremities. – Keep follow-up appointment and tests.
Vincristine	• Peripheral neuropathy • Constipation • Alopecia • Paralytic Ileus • Jaw pain • Foot drop	—	• Constipation – Sit upright when having a bowel movement. – Do not try to "hold" passing stool. – Drink 8–10 or more glasses of fluid daily. – Drink a warm or hot drink 30 minutes before bedtime. – Eat foods high in fiber. – Exercise daily. – Take prescribed medications to prevent constipation.

(Continued on next page)

Table 21-3. Patient Education for Part 1 of Hyper-CVAD Regimen *(Continued)*

Chemotherapy	Side Effects	Immediate Patient Education	Discharge Patient Education
Vincristine *(cont.)*			• Peripheral neuropathy – Report loss of sensation, numbness, and tingling to healthcare provider. • Secondary malignancy – Understand importance of keeping follow-up appointments.
Cyclophospha-mide	• Hemorrhagic cystitis • Vomiting • Dose-limiting myelo-suppression • Nausea • Alopecia • Secondary malignancy • Testicular or ovarian failure	• Instruct patient to be well hydrated and to void frequently. • Instruct patient about risk for nausea and vomiting (see information under doxorubicin).	

Note. Based on information from Callaghan & Cooper, 2014; Caplinger et al., 2010; Haylock et al., 2014; Oncology Nursing Society, 2014; Polovich et al., 2014; Shelton, 2009a; Zitella et al., 2009.

- Cytarabine (1,500 mg/m^2) 3,060 mg IV over two hours every 12 hours on days 2 and 3
- Leucovorin 15 mg IVPB over 15 minutes every 6 hours on days 3 and 4; critical to begin 24 hours after completion of methotrexate infusion
- Filgrastim 480 mcg SC on days 5–11.

The nurse will provide J.B. with antiemetics to prevent nausea and vomiting; steroid eye drops for use before, during, and after cytarabine; and antimicrobials to prevent infection. The nurse will also perform a neurologic check before each dose of cytarabine.

Table 21-4. Pretreatment Laboratory Values, Part 2	
Test	Laboratory Value
White blood cell count	9.6/mm^3
Red blood cell count	3.46 million/mcl (low)
Hemoglobin	11.2 g/dl (low)
Hematocrit	35.6% (low)
Platelet count	283,000/mm^3
Segmented neutrophils	68.6% (high)
Bands	0%
Absolute neutrophil count	6,586/mm^3
Sodium	140 mEq/L
Potassium	4.0 mEq/L
Chloride	105 mEq/L
Carbon dioxide	7 mEq/L
Blood urea nitrogen	21 mg/dl
Glucose	121 mg/dl
Calcium	8.6 mg/dl
Phosphate	2.9 mg/dl
Albumin	3.3 g/dl
Lactate dehydrogenase	204 U/L

J.B. will be instructed to report any mental status changes, gait problems, or other neurologic changes and to wear sunscreen with sun protection factor of 15 or greater, a hat, long sleeves, pants, and sunglasses. Hand hygiene and other methods to reduce risk of infection will be reinforced. See Table 21-5 for additional patient education.

Key Points

- An accurate basic physical assessment, including in-depth neurologic assessment and review of pertinent laboratory findings prior to administering chemotherapy, is essential.
- Patient should be monitored closely for tumor lysis syndrome.
- Thorough patient education includes verbal and written instructions, as well as continual reinforcement of important concepts such as infection prevention.

Conclusion

J.B. is a 64-year-old man with ALL who was discharged with appropriate patient education after receiving one course of hyper-CVAD. Overall, he tolerated the therapy well, achieved remission, and did not develop significant side effects. He will have his laboratory values checked twice weekly until he returns in three weeks to start the next course of hyper-CVAD.

References

American Cancer Society. (2015). *Cancer facts and figures 2015*. Retrieved from http://www.cancer.org/acs/groups/content/@research/documents/webcontent/acspc-042151.pdf.

Brown, C. (2010). Cerebellar assessment for patients receiving high-dose cytarabine: A standardized approach to nursing assessment and documentation. *Clinical Journal of Oncology Nursing, 14,* 371–373. doi:10.1188/10.CJON.371-373

Callaghan, M., & Cooper, A. (2014). Alopecia. In C.H. Yarbro, D. Wujcik, & B.H. Gobel (Eds.), *Cancer symptom management* (4th ed., pp. 495–505). Burlington, MA: Jones & Bartlett Learning.

Table 21-5. Patient Education for Part 2 of Hyper-CVAD

Chemotherapy	Side Effects	Immediate Patient Education	Discharge Patient Education

Methotrexate (drug is yellow in color)	• Myelosuppression
	• Nausea and vomiting
	• Mucositis
	• Photosensitivity
	• Neurotoxicity with high-dose methotrexate
		• Nausea and vomiting: See Table 21-3.
		• Mucositis: See Table 21-3.
			• Photosensitivity
			  – Wear hat and sunscreen with sun protection factor of 15 or higher.
			  – Wear sunglasses.
			• Myelosuppression: See Table 21-3.
			• Drug-drug interactions
			  – Ensure that patients do not take multivitamins with folic acid.

High-dose cytarabine	• Myelosuppression
	• Cerebellar toxicity
	• Keratitis
	• Mucositis
	• Nausea and vomiting
	• Diarrhea
	• Dermatologic toxicities
		• Cerebellar toxicity
		  – Healthcare team will perform neurologic check, including presence of nystagmus, prior to starting cytarabine and prior to each dose.
		  – Test handwriting prior to first dose to use as comparison.
		• Keratitis
		  – Patient will receive prednisolone acetate 1% eye drops to both eyes as ordered.
			• Myelosuppression: See Table 21-3.

Note. Based on information from Brown, 2010; Polovich et al., 2014.

Caplinger, J., Royse, M., & Martens, J. (2010). Implementation of an oral care protocol to promote early detection and management of stomatitis. *Clinical Journal of
Oncology Nursing, 14,* 799–802. doi:10.1188/10.CJON.799-802

Handy, C.M., Olsen, M., & Zitella, L.J. (2013). Precursor lymphoid neoplasms. In M.
Olsen & L.J. Zitella (Eds.), *Hematologic malignancies in adults* (pp. 157–200). Pittsburgh, PA: Oncology Nursing Society.

Haylock, P.J., Curtiss, C., & Massey, R.L. (2014). Constipation. In C.H. Yarbro, D.
Wujcik, & B.H. Gobel (Eds.), *Cancer symptom management* (4th ed., pp. 161–183).
Burlington, MA: Jones & Bartlett Learning.

Kurtin, S.E. (2011). Leukemia and myelodysplastic syndrome. In C.H. Yarbro, D.
Wujcik, & B.H. Gobel (Eds.), *Cancer nursing: Principles and practice* (7th ed., pp.
1369–1398). Burlington, MA: Jones & Bartlett Learning.

National Cancer Institute. (2014). Adult acute lymphoblastic leukemia treatment (PDQ®): General information about adult acute lymphoblastic leukemia
(ALL). Retrieved from http://www.cancer.gov/cancertopics/pdq/treatment/
adultALL/HealthProfessional

Oncology Nursing Society. (2014). Putting evidence into practice. Retrieved from
https://www.ons.org/practice-resources/pep

Polovich, M., Olsen, M., & LeFebvre, K.B. (Eds.). (2014). *Chemotherapy and biotherapy guidelines and recommendations for practice* (4th ed.). Pittsburgh, PA: Oncology
Nursing Society.

Shelton, B.K. (2009a). Myelosuppression. In B.H. Gobel, S. Triest-Robertson, & W.H.
Vogel (Eds.), *Advanced oncology nursing certification review and resource manual* (pp.
405–442). Pittsburgh, PA: Oncology Nursing Society.

Shelton, B.K. (2009b). Tumor lysis syndrome. In C.C. Chernecky & K. Murphy-Ende
(Eds.), *Acute care oncology nursing* (2nd ed., pp. 545–559). St. Louis, MO: Elsevier
Saunders.

Wilson, B.J., Ahmed, F., Crannell, C.E., Crego, W., Erb, C.H., Foster, J., ... Zitella, L. (2014).
Putting evidence into practice: Prevention of infection: General. Retrieved from
https://www.ons.org/practice-resources/pep/prevention-infection/prevention
-infection-general

Zitella, L.J. (2014). Infection. In C.H. Yarbro, D. Wujcik, & B.H. Gobel (Eds.), *Cancer symptom management* (4th ed., pp. 131–157). Burlington, MA: Jones & Bartlett
Learning.

Zitella, L.J., Gobel, B.H., O'Leary, C., & Belansky, H. (2009). Prevention of infection.
In L.H. Eaton & J.M. Tipton (Eds.), *Putting evidence into practice: Improving oncology
patient outcomes* (pp. 273–283). Pittsburgh, PA: Oncology Nursing Society.

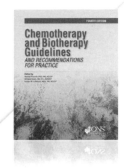

CHEMOTHERAPY AND BIOTHERAPY GUIDELINES AND RECOMMENDATIONS FOR PRACTICE (FOURTH EDITION)
Edited by M. Polovich, M. Olsen, and K. LeFebvre

Make sure you have the most up-to-date knowledge on chemotherapy, biotherapy, and targeted agents with the fourth edition of the trusted and best-selling resource *Chemotherapy and Biotherapy Guidelines and Recommendations for Practice*. Featuring revised and reorganized text, the book will help you

- Quickly and easily find information on antineoplastic therapy, post-treatment care, competencies in chemotherapy administration, and chemotherapy sequencing.
- Ensure you are up to date on the nursing management of treatment side effects.
- Improve patient education in your practice, thanks to expanded information on its importance in patient care.

Add this title to your medical library today. 2014. 473 pages. Spiral bound.

ISBN: 9781935864332 • Item: INPU0640

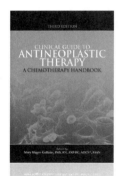

CLINICAL GUIDE TO ANTINEOPLASTIC THERAPY: A CHEMOTHERAPY HANDBOOK (THIRD EDITION)
Edited by M.M. Gullatte

The *Clinical Guide to Antineoplastic Therapy: A Chemotherapy Handbook* is an essential chemotherapy reference for clinicians at every level—from students to the most seasoned nurses involved in the care of patients receiving chemotherapy. Newly updated, revised, and expanded, the third edition will help you

- Access up-to-date, comprehensive information on antineoplastic therapy with an easy-to-use A–Z guide of more than 150 chemotherapy, biotherapy, and hormonal therapy agents.
- Confidently address the wide-ranging care issues of this patient population with chapters on patient and family support, late effects of chemotherapy, stem cell transplantation practice, strategies for improving patient adherence to chemotherapy, and survivorship.

Make sure you have the latest knowledge on antineoplastic therapy with this third edition. 2014. 1,013 pages. Softcover.

ISBN: 9781935864318 • Item: INPU0634

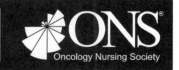